RENAL AND UROLOGIC DISORDERS

UROLITHIASIS

SYMPTOMS, MANAGEMENT AND PREVENTION STRATEGIES

RENAL AND UROLOGIC DISORDERS

Additional books in this series can be found on Nova's website under the Series tab.

Additional e-books in this series can be found on Nova's website under the e-book tab.

RENAL AND UROLOGIC DISORDERS

UROLITHIASIS

SYMPTOMS, MANAGEMENT AND PREVENTION STRATEGIES

JOSEPH FLETCHER
EDITOR

New York

Library of Congress Cataloging-in-Publication Data

ISBN: 978-1-63463-500-4

Library of Congress Control Number: 2014955172

Published by Nova Science Publishers, Inc. † New York

Contents

Preface

Urolithiasis is one of the oldest documented medical ailments with archeological evidence showing that humans have suffered from kidney and bladder stones for centuries. Urolithiasis is a common multifactorial problem with multi-effect on the patients' quality of life and an economic burden on the individual and the health system of the country. Various intrinsic and extrinsic factors are associated with the risk for stone formation. Among intrinsic factors are race, sex, and genetics. Finding the cause of urolithiasis or establishing it early in life will reduce the consequence and complications of kidney stone disease and hence reduction of the cost in the treatment by establishing preventative measures in addition to patient education. Genetic factors play an important role in the etiology of urolithiasis as a polygenic (common) or monogenic (rare) forms, however its knowledge and early diagnosis is important for achieving the goals of reducing patient suffering as well as economic burdens that inevitably follow a diagnosis. This book discusses the symptoms, management and prevention strategies of urolithiasis.

Chapter 1 – Metallic ureteral stents are one option for managing a chronically obstructed ureter. Various types of metallic stents exist and have been in use for over 15 years. The primary advantage of metallic stents over traditional polymer stents is that metallic stents have a longer approved dwell time and theoretically can be changed less frequently than polymer stents. Other benefits may be greater convenience for patients, mitigation of risks related to stent changes, and increased cost effectiveness. In this chapter the authors review the history of the metallic stent ranging from its conception to its contemporary use in clinical urologic practice. Different types of metallic stents are discussed including expandable mesh and occluded-end types of stents. Outcomes and complication reports of contemporary series are reviewed in detail. The authors finish by offering a current clinical perspective on the use of indwelling double-pigtail metallic stents, with regard to indications, patient selection, and follow-up care.

Chapter 2 – Upper tract nephrolithiasis is a common surgical condition and is treated with multiple surgical techniques including shock wave lithotripsy (SWL), ureteroscopy (URS) and percutaneous nephrolithotomy (PCNL). As more treatment modalities become available for treatment of upper tract calculi, there is a corollary increase in the complexity of decision-making in the management of these stones. Urologists are often faced with surgical scenarios in which several different treatment modalities may be acceptable and several studies have confirmed there is considerable variation in the practice patterns of urologists today. In the following chapter the authors describe the current literature and focus in detail on contemporary studies utilizing various study databases including the Medicare claims database, American Board of Urology case logs, and various administrative and surgical outcomes databases to provide a better understanding of current practice patterns of urologist globally. Overall, in the last decade, clinicians have exhibited a dramatic adoption of endoscopic techniques with a significant rise in the use of ureteroscopy and decline in the use of SWL. The treatment of upper tract calculi remains an evolving field and provider-specific attributes continue to affect how these stones are treated.

Chapter 3 – With growing socioeconomic pressure on the health systems worldwide, there is an ever growing need for efficient delivery of care with the best possible results and minimal complications. In the field of Urology and stone disease in particular, shockwave lithotripsy has revolutionized the way lithiasis is managed. The latest development involves the delivery of shockwaves into the acutely obstructing ureteric stone in the form of emergency lithotripsy (eSWL). It allows for rapid pain relief and stone expulsion, thereby reducing morbidity, operating lists waiting times and time off work.

In this chapter, the authors shall describe the principles of shockwave lithotripsy in brief, as well as the indications and contraindications, as a prelude to the more specialized circumstances of emergency lithotripsy. They will outline the basic pathophysiologic principles behind emergency treatment and the evidence behind the evolution of a dedicated protocol that produces excellent results in the context of day case treatment. The authors will also describe a referral pathway specifically designed to funnel patients into the service within a specified time frame suitable for the application of emergency shockwave treatment.

Chapter 4 – Urolithiasis is a common multifactorial problem with multi-effect on the patients' quality of life and an economic burden on the individual and the health system of the country. Various intrinsic and extrinsic factors are associated with the risk for stone formation. Among intrinsic factors are race, sex, and genetics. Finding the cause of urolithiasis or establishing it early in life will reduce the consequence and complications of kidney stone disease and hence reduction of the cost in the treatment by establishing preventative measures in addition to patient education. Genetic factors play an important role in the etiology of urolithiasis as a polygenic (common) or monogenic (rare) forms, however its knowledge and early diagnosis is important to achieve the goals of reducing patient suffering and the economic burdens. This chapter entitled "Hereditary Kidney Stones" is devoted to understanding, early recognition, management and prevention of complications of hereditary urolithasis. This topic is important for urologists in practice to have an in depth knowledge about hereditary kidney stones and how to evaluate and manage them in addition to counseling the patients and their families.

Chapter 5 – The management of paediatric stone disease has undergone a dramatic evolution in recent times. Over the past two decades, surgical management of urolithiasis in children has developed significantly. Shock wave lithotripsy (SWL) is currently the procedure of choice in treating most upper tract calculi in paediatric urolithiasis. In a growing number of centres, the use of ureteroscopy (URS) has dramatically increased, and is now the first choiceapproach for upper tract stones. Percutaneous nephrolithotomy (PCNL) has replaced open surgical techniques for the treatment of large stone burdens greater than 2 cm in size, with efficacy and complication rates similar to those of the adult population. Recently, laparoscopy and robotic techniques have become an option in the management of paediatric urolithiasis.

This chapter will focus on recent advances in the surgical management of paediatric stone disease.

Chapter Outline:

- Overview of the management of paediatric stones
- Shock wave lithotripsy
- Percutaneous nephrolithotomy
- Ureteroscopy
- Laparoscopic and robotic-assisted pyelolithotomy

In: Urolithiasis
Editor: Joseph Fletcher
ISBN: 978-1-63463-500-4

Chapter 1

Use of Metallic Stents for Chronic Ureteral Obstruction

Adam O. Kadlec[1], Arpeet Shah[1], Luke Frederick[2] and Thomas M. Turk[1]
[1]Loyola University Medical Center, Department of Urology
Maywood, IL, US
[2]Southern Illinois University School of Medicine
Division of Urology, Springfield, IL, US

Abstract

Metallic ureteral stents are one option for managing a chronically obstructed ureter. Various types of metallic stents exist and have been in use for over 15 years. The primary advantage of metallic stents over traditional polymer stents is that metallic stents have a longer approved dwell time and theoretically can be changed less frequently than polymer stents.

Other benefits may be greater convenience for patients, mitigation of risks related to stent changes, and increased cost effectiveness. In this chapter we review the history of the metallic stent ranging from its conception to its contemporary use in clinical urologic practice. Different types of metallic stents are discussed including expandable mesh and occluded-end types of stents. Outcomes and complication reports of contemporary series are reviewed in detail. We finish by offering a current clinical perspective on the use of indwelling double-pigtail metallic stents, with regard to indications, patient selection, and follow-up care.

Introduction

Chronic ureteral obstruction is encountered relatively commonly in a general urologic practice, and carries with it an array of treatment options. Traditional treatment options include percutaneous nephrostomy, drainage with an indwelling ureteral stent, and formal reconstruction (e.g. pyeloplasty, ureteroneocystostomy). The purpose and scope of this chapter is a comprehensive review of one management option for chronic ureteral obstruction – the metallic ureteral stent.

Ureteral obstruction is not a uniform diagnosis and may be characterized in a number of ways. Commonly used characterizations and dichotomies include terms such as: a) benign or malignant; b) intrinsic or extrinsic; c) proximal or distal; d) high-grade or low-grade; e) anatomic or functional; f) congenital or acquired. Further sub-classification occurs even within these categories – for instance, <2cm or >2cm ureteral stricture has treatment-related implications. Special cases of ureteral obstruction may include cases seen in the pediatric population, cases related to urinary diversion, and cases that are post-operative in nature. Beyond that, there are patient-related factors that may factor into the classification and management of ureteral obstruction: age and comorbidity, prognosis and/or life span if cancer is present, uro-anatomic abnormality, body habitus, and functional status. Finally, cost concerns have come into play as cost-related outcomes come under closer scrutiny.

For these and other reasons, analysis of outcomes for any management strategy must take into account the targeted patient population; studies should be viewed in light of inclusion criteria and metrics of follow-up, as well as upon the type of management option used. These previous points also have design implications and may explain why we have seen numerous management options and iterations over the years. An ideal management option for chronic ureteral obstruction must be clinically effective, offer low rates of complication and morbidity, be cost effective – and all the while should be well-suited to any of the multiple types of ureteral obstruction that may be present in various clinical scenarios. It is no wonder that we are still awaiting a “perfect” solution for chronic ureteral obstruction.

Historical Perspectives

It is well-accepted that chronic ureteral stenting can be a problematic management strategy for chronic ureteral obstruction. Historical case series of polymer stenting have identified stent intolerance, high failure rates, costs of stent exchanges, and the short life span of patients with malignant obstruction as factors that have made chronic stenting an unfavorable although often necessary solution to ureteral obstruction [1,2]. In light of that, the search for an ideal stent has been ongoing. Theoretical advantages of metallic stents over polymer stents include but are not limited to longer approved dwell time, improved resistance to external compression [3], and perhaps increased cost-effectiveness [4,5].

The first case series of metallic stenting in the genitourinary tract was in 1988. Milroy et al., reported a case series of stainless steel self-expandable mesh metal stents (UroLume, American Medical Systems, Minnetonka, MN) placed in the *urethra* of patients with urethral stricture [6]. *Ureteral* use of metallic stents dates to the 1990s and stemmed originally from prior experience with metallic stents (or endoprostheses) in the biliary and vascular systems, which were typically mesh stents that were self- or balloon-expandable. These open-lumen expandable mesh metallic stents were the earliest models of metallic ureteral stents.

Use of mesh stents in the ureter was initially adopted by radiologists and several case series were published in the 1990s [7-10]. In 1997, Barbalias et al., reported a series of 12 patients with malignant ureteral obstruction treated with self- and balloon-expandable metallic stents. These earlier generations of metallic ureteral stents did suffer from drawbacks, most notably urothelial hyperplasia within the stent lumen. Other problems included encrustation, stent migration, and urinary infection. A more detailed analysis of these early series appears later in this chapter.

Early-generation open-lumen expandable mesh stents can be inserted via retrograde or antegrade technique, by either a urologist or a radiologist. Antibiotic prophylaxis within 24 hours of stent insertion is recommended. First, a percutaneous nephrostomy tube is placed and antegrade pyelouretrography is performed. Once the strictured or narrowed ureteral segment is identified, it is bypassed with a guidewire. The narrowed area is then dilated and the mesh stent is inserted in its place. The upper end of the stent should be 3-4 cm above the narrowed segment and the lower end should traverse the ureterovesical junction and extend about 1 cm into the bladder from the ureteral orifice. Long (>6 cm) areas of narrowing may be managed with two metallic stents in series. Stents in series should overlap by 2-3 cm. A plain film of the abdomen may be performed to confirm proper placement and the nephrostomy tube can then be removed or capped depending on the clinical scenario. Follow-up regimens are variable but most authors recommend KUB or renal US, serum Cr, and/or renography to confirm that the obstruction remains adequately treated as time progresses (adapted from Liatskos et al., *Metal Stents in the Urinary Tract*, EAU-EBU Update 2006.)

After the initial use and reported outcomes of metallic stents for patients with malignant ureteral obstruction, applicability has widened and subsequent studies have applied metallic stents to ureteroileal strictures [11,12], strictures in renal transplant patients [13,14], and other benign conditions [15].

Later iterations of expandable open-lumen stents included covered stents, which were designed to minimize tissue ingrowth and urothelial hyperplasia, and thermoexpandable stents, which were designed to self-expand under the influence of body temperature [16]. Both types of stents are placed in antegrade or retrograde fashion and may be placed across the stricture only (i.e. they need not cross the ureterovesical junction).

More recently, the Resonance® metallic stent (Cook Medical, Bloomington, IN) was FDA-approved for ureteral obstruction. The Resonance stent is an occluded-end, metal alloy, double-pigtail stent that transverses the entire ureter. The first use was reported by Borin et al., in 2006 [17]. Potential advantages of the Resonance® stent include familiar method of placement (retrograde, though it can be placed antegrade as well), ease of removal, resistance to encrustation, and improved resistance to external compression. The device is not designed to be permanent and is recommended to be exchanged at approximately one-year intervals.

Types of Metallic Stents Available for Clinical Use

Liatsikos and colleagues have previously summarized the properties of an ideal ureteral stent [18]. It should be relatively straightforward to insert, with high success and low complication rates, and have excellent long-term patency. It should be tolerable to the patient and should not degrade, encrust, or disrupt flow in the urinary tract. The stent should be visible on ultrasound and radiographic studies. As mentioned earlier, it should be well-suited for the different types of ureteral obstruction commonly encountered in clinical practice. The three types of metallic ureteral stents available for clinical use appear in Table 1. The UVENTA® and Memokath® are open-lumen mesh metal stents designed for "permanent" use, while the Resonance® is a double-pigtail indwelling stent with an approved dwell time of one year. Only the Resonance® stent is FDA-approved for use in the United States.

Table 1. The three types of metallic stents currently marketed. Only the Resonance® stent is currently available for commercial use in the United States

Name	Country of origin	Company	Composition	Description
UVENTA® ureteral stent	South Korea	Taewoong Medical Co.	Two layers of nitinol mesh with a Teflon layer in between	- Covered Self-expandable Dual-layered Metallic Mesh Stent - Undergoing phase 4 clinical trials in USA
Memokath® 051	Denmark	Pnn Medical Co.	Thermo-expandable titanium-nickel	- Spiral metal stent - 3, 6, 10, 15, or 20 lengths available - Undergoing phase 2 clinical trials in USA
Resonance® ureteral stent	USA	Cook Medical	Nickel-cobalt-chromium-molybdenum alloy	- Approved for use in benign and malignant ureteral obstruction - Approved for up to 12 months - Most well studied metal stent in the USA

The UVENTA® stent (Taewoong Medical, S. Korea) is an open-lumen triple-layer covered stent composed of two layers of nitinol with a PTFE (Teflon) membrane in between. The stent was designed to minimize tissue ingrowth and "hold" the urothelium to prevent migration [16,19]. The stent is currently undergoing Phase IV clinical trials in the United States.

The Memokath® 051 (Pnn Medical, Denmark) ureteral stent is a thermoxpandable shape-memory spiral metallic stent that is softens at lower (10 deg C) and hardens at higher (50 deg C) temperatures. Though the device is designed for long-term use, its shape memory properties allow for easier removal and/or replacement if clinically indicated. Insertion of bilateral

Memokath® 051 stents in a patient with urinary diversion has been reported [12]. 11-year outcome data were published in 2009 [20]. The stent is currently undergoing Phase II clinical trials in the United States.

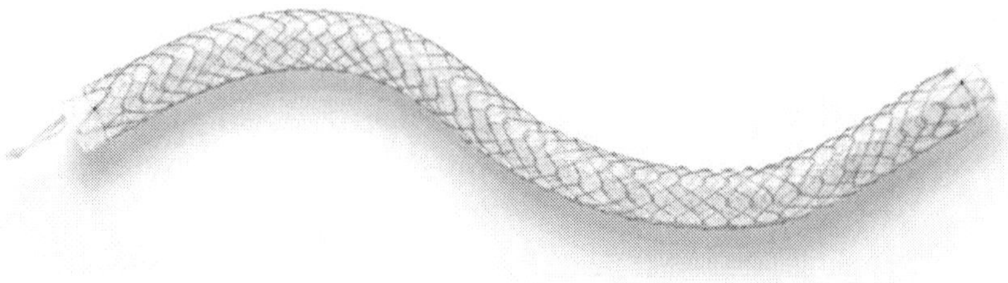

Figure 1. An image of the UVENTA™ stent.

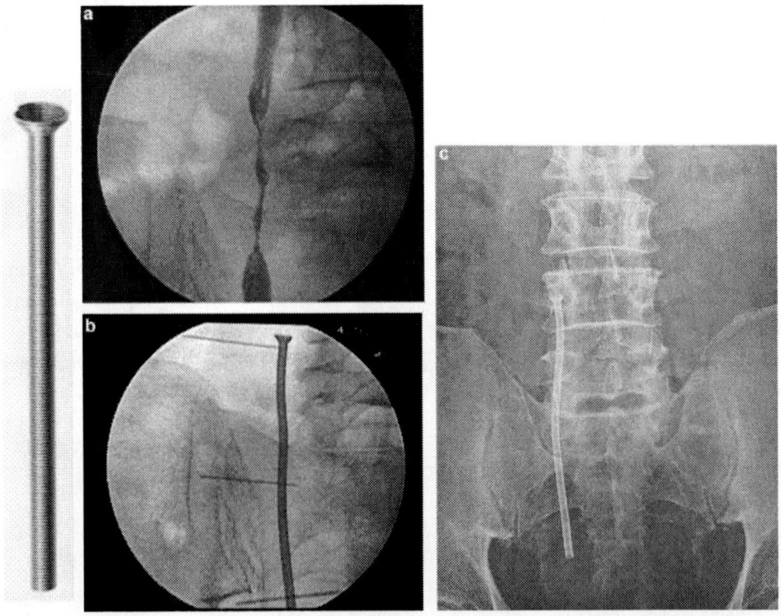

Figure 2. Images from Azizi et al. (21) depicting a schematic of the Memokath™ stent as well as representative radiographic images.

The Resonance® stent (Cook Medical, Bloomington, IN) is a 6-French occluded-end, metal alloy, double-pigtail stent that transverses the entire ureter. The first use was reported by Borin et al., in 2006 [17].

Five-year outcome data were published in 2013 [22]. Potential advantages of the Resonance® stent include ease of removal, resistance to encrustation, and improved resistance to external compression.

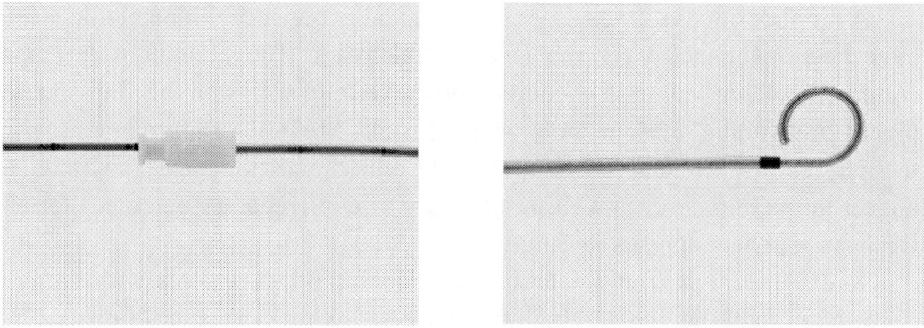

Figure 3. The Resonance® stent and its inner obturator (above) and clear plastic introducer sheath (below). Photos from Cook Medical, used with permission.

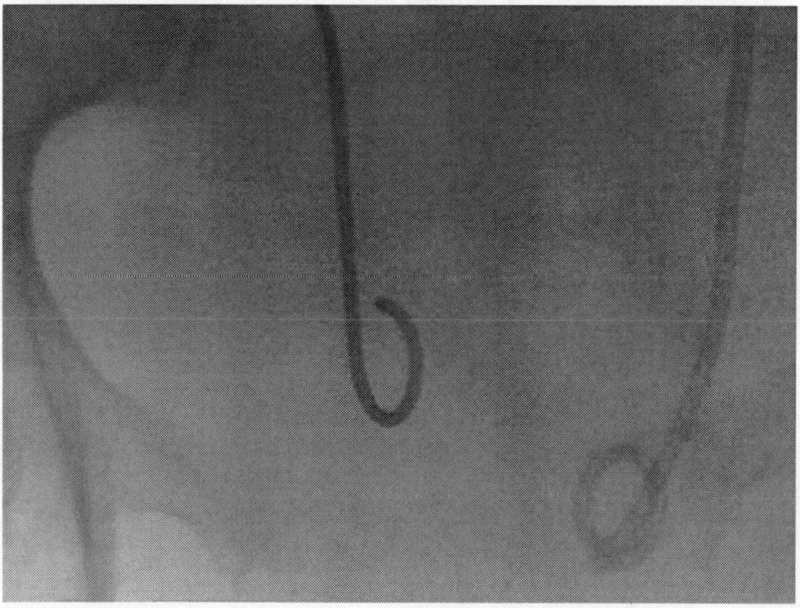

Figure 4. Note the radiographic appearance of the Resonance® stent, shown on the left in the radiograph, alongside a contralateral traditional polymer stent.

Contemporary Outcomes for Metallic Stents

A number of case series describing clinical experience with metallic stents have been published over the last several years. The metallic stent most commonly described in the contemporary setting seems to be the double-pigtail indwelling Resonance® stent (Cook Medical, Bloomington, IN), though reports on both the UVENTA® and the Memokath® continue to appear in the literature, as well. A summary of contemporary outcomes for the Resonance® stent appears in Table 1.

In 2010, Liatsikos et al., described a cohort of 50 patients with ureteral obstruction, both benign and malignant, treated with Resonance® stents [23]. Seven of the 50 patients had a previously obstructed mesh metal stent in place. 20 stents were inserted antegrade. The study was limited by a mean follow-up of 8.5 months (maximum 14 months) but it provided the first relatively large single-institution series for the Resonance® stent. One finding of particular interest was a relatively negative experience with "benign" obstruction – only eight of 18 patients with benign obstruction were successfully managed. Three of those patients had ureteroileal strictures, which over time have proved to be recalcitrant to metallic stenting (see other studies below). Four patients had extensive iatrogenic stricture. Another concern raised by the authors was stent encrustation, which developed in 12 of 54 stents. One stent in a stone-forming patient developed enough encrustation to require removal shortly after placement.

The largest clinical experience with the longest follow-up was published in 2013 by Kadlec et al. The authors described a five-year experience with Resonance® stents for benign and malignant obstruction, with 47 patients and 139 stents [22]. Mean and maximum follow-up was 20 and 59 months, respectively.

Failure (defined as any event that led to discontinuation of metallic stents as a management strategy) occurred in 28% of patients and the rate did not differ between patients with benign and malignant obstruction. Median duration of stenting was 22 months in the patients with benign obstruction and 7 months in patients with malignant obstruction. A survival curve representing duration of stenting did not differ between patients with benign and malignant obstruction when the higher death rate in the malignant group was taken into account (Figure 4).

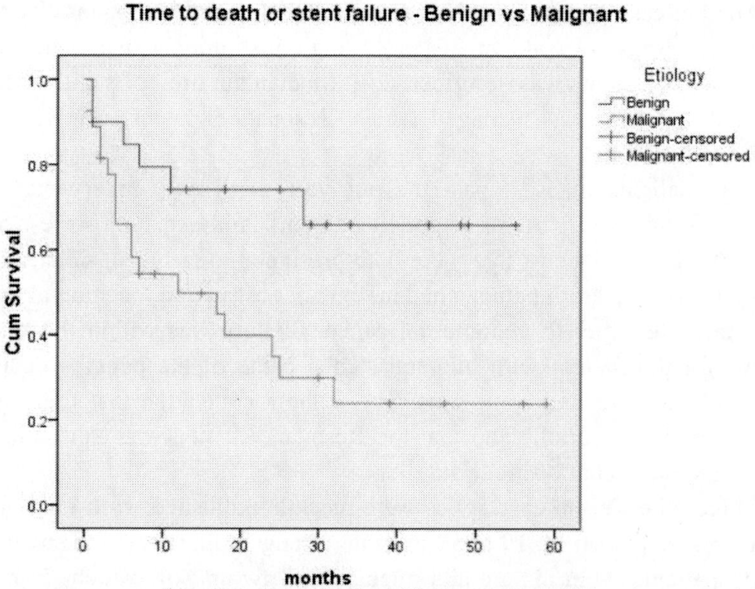

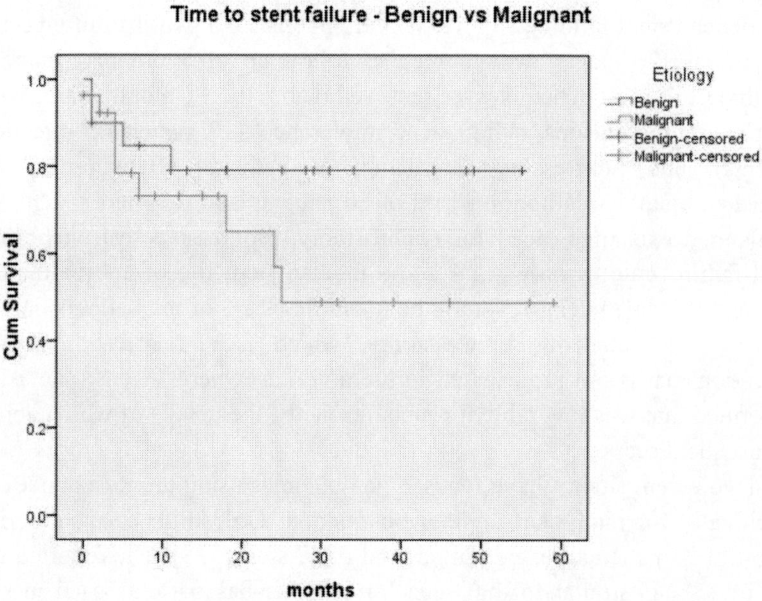

Figure 5. Kaplan-Meier curves of event-free stent retention by obstruction etiology in benign (blue curves) and malignant (green curves) groups. A, observed events were stent failure and death (benign vs malignant log rank test $p = 0.016$). B, observed event was stent failure (benign vs malignant log rank test $p = 0.178$). Cum, cumulative.

Another case series in a cohort of mixed benign and malignant obstruction came from Benson et al., in 2011. A single-institution experience with 23 patients and 42 stents was described [24]. Median duration of stenting (i.e. the time that a patient was managed with a Resonance® stent) was 13 months (range 2-32 months).

Nine patients made it past the one-year mark and underwent a stent exchange. Only two patients experienced stent failure in this series, one of whom had bilateral stents that were both presumed to fail (3 of 42 stents, or a 7.1% failure rate). Both patients had malignant obstruction, one due to prostate cancer and the other to endometrial cancer. Failure was within the first two months for the patient with bilateral stents. None of the patients developed intolerable stent-related symptoms. The authors concluded that their clinical experience was favorable and that the Resonance® stent was suited for both benign and malignant obstruction.

Three other recent case series were recently published, with total number of patients ranging from 19 to 50 patients. Wang et al., reported a small series of 19 patients with 5 months median follow-up, of which 5 patients experienced stent failure [25]. Modi et al., published a two-institution series of 40 patients (76 stents) with a median follow-up of 5 months (range 0-18 months) [26]. 43% of stents were removed before the 12-month mark, with the most common reasons being stent intolerance (10 patients), infection (8 patients), and progressive obstruction (9 patients). Baumgarten et al., published a single-institution series of 50 patients and reported a stent failure (unplanned exchange, need for nephrostomy, progressive hydronephrosis or renal failure) rate of only 8.2% and a median stent life of approximately 10 months (288 days) [27]. It should be noted that 24% of the patients had stents placed in a cutaneous ureterostomy, which is a relatively uncommon indication that is not represented in literature elsewhere. A cost analysis was performed that was favorable for metallic stents, the details of which appear in a subsequent section.

Two recent studies have focused on outcomes using the Resonance® stent specifically for malignant ureteral obstruction. Goldsmith et al., described a cohort of 25 patients treated with a total of 37 stents [28]. The reported failure rate of 35% is similar to that seen for polymer-based stents used in similar patient populations. Patients with high-grade obstruction due to locally advanced prostate cancer fared particularly poorly, and the authors reported a statistically significant increase in stent failure rates for these patients, though that finding should be interpreted with caution in light of the number of patients in the study. Three stents migrated distally and three symptomatic subcapsular hematomas occurred, which the authors suggest may have been related to the inner cannula of the introducer system protruding well beyond the radio-opaque marker located on the outer sheath that is often used to judge the extent of proximal insertion. More recently, Abbasi et al., published on a cohort of 20 patients (27 stents) with malignant ureteral obstruction. In this series, eight of the 20 patients required a secondary intervention (i.e. 40% failure rate) and the mean time to failure was 7.4 months. Two patients were converted to nephrostomy drainage, four were converted to polymer stents, and two simply had their stents removed. The study period ran from mid-2007 to mid-2009 and at the time of last follow-up, presumably around the time of publication in 2013, 16 of the 20 patients had died, 14 with functional stents in place [29].

Some groups have published data pertaining to relatively specific clinical situations. Lang et al., described a series of 24 patients with malignant ureteral obstruction secondary to cervical carcinoma (stage T3b or T4) that was treated with Wallstents®. Placement was successful in all patients, and the authors report 18-month patency in 54% of patients, although it appears that a significant number of secondary procedures (i.e., laser ablation of obstructing intraluminal tissue) were required to achieve continued patency [30]. Gayed et al., reported a negative experience with Resonance® stents in two pediatric patients, the first of which experienced stent failure at three months and the other at two weeks. The title of the article suggests that the authors have deemed metallic stenting unfit for pediatric patients, though the fact that both patients ultimately required extensive urologic reconstruction makes one wonder if stent failure occurred due to nature of disease rather than pediatric patient selection [31]. Two recent studies reported on the successful use of metallic stents in renal transplant patients – one being a 12-cm x 6-Fr Resonance® stent in a single transplanted kidney [13] and the other a series of eight male transplant patients treated with Memokath® stents. Half of those stents remained functional at mean follow-up of 4.5 years. Finally, Garg et al., reported on a series of ten ureteroileal strictures treated with Resonance® stents, nine of which migrated distally within 60 days [32]. This data strongly suggests that Resonance® stents are not an appropriate management strategy for ureteroileal strictures. A more favorable experience on ureteroileal stricture management comes from Al-Mahmid et al., though they report on only a single patient and a Memokath® stent was used [12].

An ongoing clinical issue is preoperative identification of factors that may adversely affect the success rate of metallic stenting.

Table 2. Contemporary clinical outcomes for the Resonance® stent

First Author	Date	n	Mean/Median Follow-up	Obstruction type	Notable findings
Chow	2014	79	4-476 days	100% malignant	- Functional duration was 5.77 mos - 65% 3 month patency rate - 44% 6 month patency rate - Age, preoperative creatinine level, and lower gastrointestinal cancers were independent risk factors for stent failure in multivariate analysis
Kadlec	2013	47	20 months	57% malignant 43% benign	- 28% stent failure rate - Stenting duration 22 mos (malignant) vs. 7 mos (benign), equivalent when corrected for death rate
Abbasi	2013	20	12 months	100% malignant	- 7.4 mos to stent failure - 40% required further intervention for obstruction - 10% required nephrostomy tube placement
Goldsmith	2012	25	11 months	100% malignant	- 35% stent failure rate - Invasion of prostate cancer into bladder significantly increases risk of failure
Benson	2011	23	12 months		- No early discontinuation for stent related symptoms or complications - 7.3% stent failure rate - Stent failure was only seen in malignant obstruction group
Modi	2010	40	5 months	19% benign 81% malignant	- 37% stent failure rate - 14% required stent removal for stent symptoms
Liatsikos	2010	50	8.5 months	50% malignant 36% benign 14% Failed metal mesh stent	- 100% stricture patency in malignant obstruction group at 11 mos - 44% stricture patency in benign obstruction group at 6.8 mos - All failed in those with previous mesh metal stent - 12% had gross hematuria that resolved spontaneously

Factors such as history of radiation and type of malignancy have been studied, with variable results and conclusions [22, 28, 33]. While some clinical scenarios clearly portend a poor outcome with metallic stents (e.g. patients with uretero-enteric strictures), it is probably safe to say that no historical or "patient-related" factor has been definitively identified as adverse with regard to clinical outcomes.

Complications of Metallic Stenting

The most commonly cited complications of metallic stenting are urinary tract infection, hematuria, progressive renal failure, and stent intolerance. Less commonly reported complications are subcapsular hematoma [28], distal migration [26], irritative LUTS [34], and stent encrustation [23]. Intraluminal proliferation of tissue is a complication that is specific to open-lumen mesh stents (such as the UVENTA® and Memokath®). It can be treated with Holmium laser ablation [30].

Knowledge of potential complications is important for both patient counseling as well as clinical management, as the literature shows that most reported complications lead to discontinuation of metallic stents as a management strategy. As the design of metallic stents evolves, it is likely that prevention of these management-ending complications will be emphasized.

Table 3. Common complications in four large series using the Resonance® stent. Progressive renal failure defined as increase in serum Cr and/or increasing hydronephrosis on imaging [NR = not reported]

First Author, Year	Urinary tract infection *(n, % total patients or stents)*	Progressive renal failure *(n, % total patients or stents)*	Gross hematuria *(n, % total patients or stents)*
Liatsikos, 2010	4, *8% of patients*	14, *28% of patients*	6, *12% of patients*
Modi, 2010	NR	19, *35% of patients*	NR
Goldsmith, 2011	0, *0% of stents*	12, *35% of stents*	NR
Kadlec, 2013	7, *5% of stents*	5, *11% of patients*	1

Economics of Metallic Stenting

One of the more common criticisms of metallic stents is that their cost is not justified for malignant obstruction, given the combination of relatively high failure rates, costs associated with stent-related complications, and short life span of patients with advanced malignancy [28]. A handful of studies have attempted to address this concern thorough simple cost analysis – all have used the Resonance® stent.

Metallic stent cost is variable but the cost of a Resonance® is approximated at $800-1,000. Polymer stents cost approximately $100. Proponents of metallic stents believe that the cost savings attributable to less frequent stent changes (and the attendant fees of stent exchange) make up for the cost of the stent itself, even though the stent itself is more expensive. Whether or not the stent is more cost-effective than a nephrostomy tube remains an unstudied, and perhaps more philosophical, question.

In 2010, Lopez-Huertas et al., analyzed 15 stents initially placed in 13 patients [34]. Management with metallic stents was discontinued in three patients (two for LUTS and one for hematuria). Eight patients underwent a stent exchange at a mean time of approximately 12 months. The yearly costs for metallic stent use in a given patient were $11,183 versus $23,999 for polymer stents, with the majority of cost savings attributable to avoidance of the fees associated with stent exchange itself.

Taylor et al., performed a direct cost description based on their retrospective experience. In the Taylor study, direct charges were tabulated in 21 patients [5]. Mean charges were $9,469.50 and $6,072.75 for the metallic and polymer stent exchanges, respectively. Under the assumption that polymer stents would need to changed more frequently than metallic stents (3-6 times per year compared to 1-2 times per year), the authors concluded that metallic stents may be considered financially advantageous in properly selected patients. Though the study did use "real-world" cost data, it was limited by the fact that it did not take actual observed outcomes (for instance, mean dwell times for metallic stents) into account when comparing costs.

Baumgarten et al., included a cost analysis in their retrospective study of 50 patients. Only patients with malignant obstruction (74% of the cohort) were analyzed. In that series, a metallic stent had a mean dwell time, or "life" of 0.79 years and a polymer stent was presumed to have a life of 0.25 years. Based on a cost of $3,327 for metallic stent placement and $2,412 for polymer stent placement, management with metallic stents provided a cost savings of over $5,000 annually [27]. The authors acknowledged some limitations of their analysis, one of which was the lack of follow-up costs such as repeat procedures, subsequent admissions, and follow-up imaging.

In summary, the cost-effectiveness studies to date have been relatively simple and somewhat more conceptual than "real-life". That being said, it is reasonable to assume that metallic stenting is probably financially advantageous over polymer stent changes if mean dwell times are consistently longer for metallic stents. Proper patient selection has a large impact on mean dwell times and therefore has major cost implications. Whether or not metallic stents are more cost-effective than nephrostomy tubes has not been studied. In any event, the cost-effectiveness of metallic stenting remains an open issue and a larger, more broadly applicable, and a more finely tuned cost analysis on the subject would be an excellent addition to the literature.

Table 4. A summary of three studies that have performed simple comparative cost analysis between metal and polymer stents. All studies used Resonance® stents

First Author	Year	N	Etiology	Notable findings
Taylor	2012	21	67% benign 33% malignant	- 48-74% cost reduction using metal stents
Lopez-Huertas	2010	13	100% benign	- 43% cost reduction using metal stents
Baumgarten	2014	50	100% malignant (benign excluded from analysis)	- approximately 57% cost reduction using metal stents

Current Clinical Perspectives on the Resonance® Metallic Stent

In this section, we offer our clinical perspective on use of the double-pigtail indwelling (Resonance®) metallic stent.

Indications, Alternatives, and Risks

Patients with chronic ureteral obstruction and anatomy that is amenable to indwelling stent placement may be considered for a Resonance® stent. Alternatives include watchful waiting, nephrostomy tube drainage, placement of a polymer-based stent, or formal reconstruction. Patients should be informed of common risks of the procedure, which include urinary tract infection, injury to the ureter or collecting system, and stent migration. Complications of stenting such as stent intolerance, hematuria, and recurrent infection should also be discussed. Both the patient and clinician should expect stent exchange after approximately 12 months.

Patient Selection

Patients with chronic ureteral obstruction who are not candidates for formal reconstruction can be considered for metallic stent placement. The bulk of the literature suggests that clinical outcomes are similar whether or not patients have benign (typically intrinsic) or malignant (typically extrinsic) obstruction. Some experts advocate for an initial trial of a polymer stent, though our experience suggests that many patients may be treated "up-front" with metallic stents, whether it be conversion from nephrostomy to indwelling stent, or initial stent placement in a previously un-instrumented obstructed system.

Our experience and the literature to date suggests that poor candidates for the Resonance® include but are not limited to: pediatric patients, patients with ureteroenteric strictures, patients with hemorrhagic cystitis or refractory hematuria, patients with recurrent urinary tract infections, patients at risk for ureterovascular fistula, and patients with a life expectancy certain to be less than 4 months. Some patients with distal ureteral obstruction due to locally advanced prostate cancer seem to fare poorly; we believe that these patients may be considered a population at high risk for failure but a trial of stenting is not unreasonable.

Operative Technique

Most urologists will prefer retrograde stent placement for avoidance of nephrostomy and anatomical familiarity. After cystoscopic identification and cannulation of the ureteral orifice, a PTFE wire should be passed into the renal pelvis under fluoroscopic guidance. During stent exchange, a hydrophilic wire may be passed alongside the existing stent and exchanged for a PTFE wire prior to stent removal. Ureteral length (from UPJ to UVJ) may be measured with an open-ended catheter, if necessary. The collecting system should then be opacified. Some authors [23] have reported ureteral balloon dilation prior to stent insertion. This may be beneficial for strictures treated *de novo* but is probably unnecessary in most routine placements.

The coaxial introducer system is then introduced. One must be cognizant of the additional length of the inner obturator that stretches ~3 cm beyond the radio-opaque marker at the tip of the outer sheath. If the patient has a small renal pelvis, the inner obturator may be drawn back 1-2 cm prior to insertion of the system.

In cases of tight stricture or difficult anatomy, an alternative approach is to "back-load" a rigid cystoscope over the initially placed PTFE guidewire. This allows insertion of the introducer system – and ultimately the stent – under direct vision and may prevent curling of the wire and introducer system in the bladder. This may be the preferred approach for novice users and/or those at training institutions.

The radio-opaque marker should then be advanced under live fluoroscopy until it is just beyond the level of the ureteropelvic junction. The inner obturator and guidewire are then removed as the outer sheath is held in place. The metallic stent itself is then inserted into the outer sheath and advanced under fluoroscopy (or under direct vision if a backloading technique was used) with the inner obturator of the introducer system. Once the stent is in appropriate position, it is held in place with the inner obturator while the outer sheath is withdrawn. Stent placement should be confirmed with fluoroscopy.

Follow-Up Care

Patients are typically followed with a combination of non-invasive imaging (usually ultrasound of the kidneys), measurement of serum creatinine, and periodic clinical assessment for problematic symptoms such as pain, hematuria, or bothersome voiding symptoms. Intervals of follow-up may be spaced out if the patient is doing well with the stent. Anecdotally, some patients with recurrent infections, hematuria, or stent intolerance may do well with exchange for another metallic stent of a smaller size (i.e. length). Other patients' symptoms will only abate after conversion to polymer-based stents or nephrostomy tubes. Our opinion is that a different size of metallic stent may be attempted in patients experiencing mild symptoms.

Future Directions

Basic science research on metallic ureteral stents is ongoing. One study found that paclitaxel-eluting metal mesh stents generated less mucosal hyperplasia than standard stents in pig ureters [35]. Another group is testing a hybrid covered metallic ureteral stent in a pig model [36,37]. The hybrid stent is a self-expanding internally covered mesh metal stent in which each end of the stent is free of metal mesh, which allows for a smoother transition between the central metallic body and the healthy ureter. (It is at this transition point where urothelial hyperplasia often occurs.) Initial results appear favorable. Other authors have compared the resistance to extrinsic compression among newer stent models and found favorable results for the Snake metallic stent (Prosurg Inc, San Jose, CA) [3]. Hopefully work will continue and solutions will be offered that will allow broadening of clinical applicability and minimization of stent-related complications and problems.

Conclusion

Ureteral stenting remains a common method of treatment for chronic ureteral obstruction. The body of literature on metallic stents continues to expand and use of metallic stents has increased, though remains far exceeded by use of polymer stents. Clinical outcomes for metallic stents seem comparable to polymer stents. The Resonance® stent is the only metallic stent currently FDA-approved for ureteral use in the United States. As with any urologic tool, the art of patient selection remains the primary driver of patient outcomes.

The authors declare no disclosures or conflicts of interest.

References

[1] Chung HH, Kim MD, Won JY, Won JH, Cho SB, Seo TS, et al. Multicenter experience of the newly designed covered metallic ureteral stent for malignant ureteral occlusion: comparison with double J stent insertion. *Cardiovasc Intervent Radiol.* 2014 Apr;37(2):463-470.

[2] Chung SY, Stein RJ, Landsittel D, Davies BJ, Cuellar DC, Hrebinko RL, et al. 15-Year Experience with the Management of Extrinsic Ureteral Obstruction with Indwelling Ureteral Stents. *J. Urol.* 2004 Aug;172(2):592-595.

[3] Hendlin K, Korman E, Monga M. New metallic ureteral stents: improved tensile strength and resistance to extrinsic compression. *J. Endourol.* 2012 Mar;26(3):271-274.

[4] Polcari AJ, Hugen CM, Lopez-Huertas HL, Turk TM. Cost analysis and clinical applicability of the Resonance metallic ureteral stent. *Expert Rev Pharmacoecon Outcomes Res.* 2010 Feb;10(1):11-15.

[5] Taylor ER, Benson AD, Schwartz BF. Cost analysis of metallic ureteral stents with 12 months of follow-up. *J. Endourol.* 2012 Jul;26(7):917-921.

[6] Milroy EJ, Chapple CR, Cooper JE, Eldin A, Wallsten H, Seddon AM, et al. A new treatment for urethral strictures. *Lancet* 1988 Jun 25;1(8600):1424-1427.

[7] Lugmayr HF, Pauer W. Wallstents for the treatment of extrinsic malignant ureteral obstruction: midterm results. *Radiology* 1996 Jan;198(1):105-108.

[8] vanSonnenberg E, D'Agostino HB, O'Laoide R, Donaldson J, Sanchez RB, Hoyt A, et al. Malignant ureteral obstruction: treatment with metal stents--technique, results, and observations with percutaneous intraluminal US. *Radiology* 1994 Jun;191(3):765-768.

[9] Flueckiger F, Lammer J, Klein GE, Hausegger K, Lederer A, Szolar D, et al. Malignant ureteral obstruction: preliminary results of treatment with metallic self-expandable stents. *Radiology* 1993 Jan;186(1):169-173.

[10] Lopez-Martinez RA, Singireddy S, Lang EK. The use of metallic stents to bypass ureteral strictures secondary to metastatic prostate cancer: experience with 8 patients. *J. Urol.* 1997 Jul;158(1):50-53.

[11] Liatsikos EN, Kagadis GC, Karnabatidis D, Katsanos K, Papathanassiou Z, Constantinides C, et al. Application of self-expandable metal stents for ureteroileal anastomotic strictures: long-term results. *J. Urol.* 2007 Jul;178(1):169-173.

[12] Al-Mahmid M, Ahrens U, Zimmer S, Winand S, Ozgur E, Engelmann UH, et al. Two thermoformable spiral metallic ureteral stents in a patient with ileal conduit and distal stenosis of the ureters. *Urol. Int.* 2013;90(2):136-138.

[13] Abdulmajed MI, Jones VW, Shergill IS. The first use of Resonance((R)) metallic ureteric stent in a case of obstructed transplant kidney. *Int. J. Surg. Case Rep.* 2014;5(7):375-377.

[14] Bach C, Kabir M, Goyal A, Malliwal R, Kachrilas S, El Howairis ME, et al. A self-expanding thermo-labile nitinol stent as minimally invasive treatment alternative for ureteric strictures in renal transplant patients. *J. Endourol.* 2013 Oct 9.

[15] Li X, He Z, Yuan J, Zeng G, He Y, Lei M. Long-term results of permanent metallic stent implantation in the treatment of benign upper urinary tract occlusion. *Int. J. Urol.* 2007 Aug;14(8):693-698.

[16] Barbalias GA, Liatsikos EN, Kalogeropoulou C, Karnabatidis D, Zabakis P, Athanasopoulos A, et al. Externally coated ureteral metallic stents: an unfavorable clinical experience. *Eur. Urol.* 2002 Sep;42(3):276-280.

[17] Borin JF, Melamud O, Clayman RV. Initial experience with full-length metal stent to relieve malignant ureteral obstruction. *J. Endourol.* 2006 May;20(5):300-304.

[18] Al-Aown A, Kyriazis I, Kallidonis P, Kraniotis P, Rigopoulos C, Karnabatidis D, et al. Ureteral stents: new ideas, new designs. *Ther. Adv. Urol.* 2010 Apr;2(2):85-92.

[19] Chung KJ, Park BH, Park B, Lee JH, Kim WJ, Baek M, et al. Efficacy and safety of a novel, double-layered, coated, self-expandable metallic mesh stent (Uventa) in malignant ureteral obstructions. *J. Endourol.* 2013 Jul;27(7):930-935.

[20] Agrawal S, Brown CT, Bellamy EA, Kulkarni R. The thermo-expandable metallic ureteric stent: an 11-year follow-up. *BJU Int.* 2009 Feb;103(3):372-376.

[21] Azizi A, Pasticier G, Benard A, Lapouge O, Ferriere JM, Ballanger P, et al. Tolerance and effectiveness of Memokath(R) 051 ureteral stents : a prospective 3 year follow-up study. *Prog. Urol.* 2012 May;22(5):266-272.

[22] Kadlec AO, Ellimoottil CS, Greco KA, Turk TM. Five-year experience with metallic stents for chronic ureteral obstruction. *J. Urol.* 2013 Sep;190(3):937-941.

[23] Liatsikos E, Kallidonis P, Kyriazis I, Constantinidis C, Hendlin K, Stolzenburg JU, et al. Ureteral obstruction: is the full metallic double-pigtail stent the way to go? *Eur. Urol.* 2010 Mar;57(3):480-486.

[24] Benson AD, Taylor ER, Schwartz BF. Metal ureteral stent for benign and malignant ureteral obstruction. *J. Urol.* 2011 Jun;185(6):2217-2222.

[25] Wang HJ, Lee TY, Luo HL, Chen CH, Shen YC, Chuang YC, et al. Application of resonance metallic stents for ureteral obstruction. *BJU Int.* 2011 Aug;108(3):428-432.

[26] Modi AP, Ritch CR, Arend D, Walsh RM, Ordonez M, Landman J, et al. Multicenter experience with metallic ureteral stents for malignant and chronic benign ureteral obstruction. *J. Endourol.* 2010 Jul;24(7):1189-1193.

[27] Baumgarten AS, Hakky TS, Carrion RE, Lockhart JL, Spiess PE. A single-institution experience with metallic ureteral stents: a cost-effective method of managing deficiencies in ureteral drainage. Int Braz *J. Urol.* 2014 Mar-Apr;40(2):225-231.

[28] Goldsmith ZG, Wang AJ, Banez LL, Lipkin ME, Ferrandino MN, Preminger GM, et al. Outcomes of Metallic Stents for Malignant Ureteral Obstruction. *J. Urol.* 2012 Jul 19.

[29] Abbasi A, Wyre HW, Ogan K. Use of full-length metallic stents in malignant ureteral obstruction. *J. Endourol.* 2013 May;27(5):640-645.

[30] Lang EK, Winer AG, Abbey-Mensah G, Anne R, Allaei A, Friedman F, et al. Long-term results of metallic stents for malignant ureteral obstruction in advanced cervical carcinoma. *J. Endourol.* 2013 May;27(5):646-651.

[31] Gayed BA, Mally AD, Riley J, Ost MC. Resonance metallic stents do not effectively relieve extrinsic ureteral compression in pediatric patients. *J. Endourol.* 2013 Feb;27(2):154-157.

[32] Garg T, Guralnick ML, Langenstroer P, See WA, Hieb RA, Rilling WS, et al. Resonance metallic ureteral stents do not successfully treat ureteroenteric strictures. *J. Endourol.* 2009 Jul;23(7):1199-201; discussion 1202.

[33] Chow PM, Hsu JS, Huang CY, Wang SM, Lee YJ, Huang KH, et al. Metallic ureteral stents in malignant ureteral obstruction: clinical factors predicting stent failure. *J. Endourol.* 2014 Jun;28(6):729-734.

[34] Lopez-Huertas HL, Polcari AJ, Acosta-Miranda A, Turk TM. Metallic ureteral stents: a cost-effective method of managing benign upper tract obstruction. *J. Endourol.* 2010 Mar;24(3):483-485.

[35] Liatsikos EN, Karnabatidis D, Kagadis GC, Rokkas K, Constantinides C, Christeas N, et al. Application of paclitaxel-eluting metal mesh stents within the pig ureter: an experimental study. *Eur. Urol.* 2007 Jan;51(1):217-223.

[36] Soria F, Morcillo E, Pamplona M, Uson J, Sanchez-Margallo FM. Evaluation in an animal model of a hybrid covered metallic ureteral stent: a new design. *Urology* 2013 Feb;81(2):458-463.

[37] Soria F, Rioja LA, Morcillo E, Martin C, Pamplona M, Sanchez FM. New combined approach in metallic ureteral stenting to avoid urothelial hyperplasia: study in swine model. *J. Urol.* 2011 May;185(5):1939-1945.

In: Urolithiasis
Editor: Joseph Fletcher

ISBN: 978-1-63463-500-4

Chapter 2

Modern Stone Management: Prevalence and Practice Patterns for Treatment of Upper Tract Calculi

Daniel T. Oberlin,* MD and Sarah C. Flury, MD
Department Of Urology, Northwestern Memorial Hospital,
Chicago, IL, US

Abstract

Upper tract nephrolithiasis is a common surgical condition and is treated with multiple surgical techniques including shock wave lithotripsy (SWL), ureteroscopy (URS) and percutaneous nephrolithotomy (PCNL). As more treatment modalities become available for treatment of upper tract calculi, there is a corollary increase in the complexity of decision-making in the management of these stones. Urologists are often faced with surgical scenarios in which several different treatment modalities may be acceptable and several studies have confirmed there is considerable variation in the practice patterns of urologists today. In the

* Corresponding Author: Daniel T. Oberlin MD; Email: Daniel-oberlin@northwestern.edu; Phone: 614-562-8233; Northwestern Memorial Hospital; 250 E Huron St; Chicago, IL 60654.

following chapter we describe the current literature and focus in detail on contemporary studies utilizing various study databases including the Medicare claims database, American Board of Urology case logs, and various administrative and surgical outcomes databases to provide a better understanding of current practice patterns of urologist globally.

Overall, in the last decade, clinicians have exhibited a dramatic adoption of endoscopic techniques with a significant rise in the use of ureteroscopy and decline in the use of SWL. The treatment of upper tract calculi remains an evolving field and provider-specific attributes continue to affect how these stones are treated.

Introduction

Urolithiasis is one of the oldest document medical ailments with archeological evidence showing that humans have suffered from kidney and bladder stones for centuries. For example, the first documentation of stone disease dates to the examination of Egyptian mummies by the English archeologist E. Smith, which revealed 5,000-year-old bladder stones at the funeral site of El Amrah, Egypt [1]. Regimens for treatment of diseases of the urinary tract, including stones, were found in the papyrus Ebers dating to 1500 BC. As early as ancient Mesopotamia there is documentation on stone tablets of the difference between soluble and insoluble bladder stones and recipes for treatment of nephrolithiasis.

In the modern era, approximately 13% of men and 7% of women will be diagnosed with a kidney stones in their lifetime [2]. The disease represents a significant burden on health care in the United States, with an estimated $5.3 billion annually in direct and indirect costs [3]. In addition, several reports have shown that the incidence of stone disease is on the rise as well. For example, Scales et al., showed that the prevalence of kidney stones in the United States is markedly higher when compared to historical records (1988–1994), and could be attributed to dietary and lifestyle factors [4]. Romero and colleagues, who explored the global prevalence and risk factors associated with stone disease, confirmed a similar worldwide increase in stone disease. The authors completed a meta-analysis of 75 peer-reviewed articles [5], showing a significantly increased prevalence, especially within aging population, in many countries including Germany, Ireland, Italy, Greece, Turkey, and the United States. Although an increase in the prevalence and annual incidence of kidney stones is clear, unfortunately, the etiology of increase is unclear. Kidney stone formation is usually due to genetic and environmental factors. Changes over such a short temporal period are therefore less likely due to genetic changes and more likely due to changes in our global environment.

With the increase in annual expenditure for stone disease, several studies have sought to determine associated risk factors. Demographic factors including age, gender, geographic region and ethnicity have all been shown to represent risk factors for stone formation [2, 6, 7]. For example, Scales et al., found that men have twice the prevalence of stone disease (10.6-12%) when compared to women (4.8-7.1%) [4]. Assessments of the contribution of race to stone risk have found that Hispanics and black patients demonstrate 40% and 63% decreased likelihood of stone disease compared to Caucasian patients [4, 8]. In a report by Stamatelou et al., [2] prevalence rates from 1976-1994 were highest among whites, followed by Hispanics, blacks, and Asians. Overall, white men have the highest rates of stone disease in the United States.

Age has also been shown to contribute to stone disease; Individuals older than 65 are more than twice as likely to have stone disease compared to middle-aged individuals 35- 49 years old [9]. Finally, geographic region has been shown to contribute to risk of stone formation. In particular, patients living in the U.S. Southeast (the stone belt) have a significantly higher incidence and prevalence of urolithiasis [10].

Not only has the prevalence of kidney stones increased in recent years, but the treatment options for surgeons have also changed. Historically, open surgical removal of kidney stones was the surgical gold standard and only option for most urologists. Yet, over the last thirty years the management of urinary tract stone disease has undergone tremendous changes. Many of these revolutions were prompted by the adoption of new technologic and treatment advances [11-14]. In the current era, open surgery has almost completely disappeared and comprises between only 0.3–4% of all stone surgery cases. According to the Urologic Diseases of America Project, rates of open surgery among commercially insured individuals decreased by half between 1992 and 2000 [15]. In the modern era, surgical intervention for stone disease includes ureteroscopy (URS), extracorporeal shock wave lithotripsy (SWL) and percutaneous nephrolithotomy (PCNL). Because of the high stone-free rates achieved with less-invasive treatments, open surgery is reserved for only the most complex stones and those with altered renal anatomy.

Although risk factors for development of stone disease have been accurately identified, studies assessing differences in treatment practice patterns are less common. As more treatment modalities become available for treatment of upper tract calculi, there is a corollary increase in the complexity of decision-making in the management of these stones. Urologists are often faced with surgical scenarios in which several different treatment modalities may be acceptable and several studies have confirmed there is considerable variation in the practice patterns of urologists today [15-17]. The emergence of this increasingly complex clinical decision-making has led us to explore contemporary surgical trends in upper tract stone management.

Until recently, only a few randomized controlled trials have been performed to determine the efficacy of various treatment options for renal stones [18, 19] and even fewer have examined surgical trends of all three modalities for stone treatment [6, 14, 20, 21]. Unfortunately, the majority of studies available are retrospective in nature and rely on limited national sampling database studies or recall-biased voluntary surveys. For example, Nakada and Colleagues completed a retrospective survey assessing practice patterns of Urologists in the North Central United States and found contemporary treatment patterns of stone disease to match the treatment approach recommended in the published literature [22]. Unfortunately, recall bias and low response rate lessen the significance of most surveys completed to date.

Ghani et al., utilized the Nationwide Inpatient Sample (NIS) to assess temporal trends in the treatment of upper urinary tract calculi in the US, but this study only examined inpatient data, whereas most kidney stone treatments are outpatient procedures [23]. Both Scales et al. and Seklehner et al., examined the utilization of SWL and URS and the effect on re-treatment rate, but did so using the medicare 5% sample, which captures data from patients 65 years of age and older, but unfortunately does not offer a complete cross-section of the patient population [6, 24].

Global assessments of stone practice patterns include those by Lee el al on the Australian patient population. The authors utilized the Australian Medicare database between 1995 and 2010 and found a dramatic increase in the use of URS and decline in SWL. Unfortunately, like many administrative databases, the study was unable to determine if the escalation in endoscopic procedures was due to an increase in the incidence of stone disease, earlier detection, a lower intervention threshold or a higher retreatment rate [25]. In the UK, Turney et al. examined treatment utilization trends and found an overall increase in the total number of stone surgeries performed, most notably that SWL use remained stable over 10 years while the use of URS more than doubled [20]. Although the study size was significant and an appropriate duration of study, all of the data was reported as a procedure count and not a rate or proportion; the data is therefore difficult to interpret, as it does not account for an increase in the UK population over the 10-year study period, nor an increase in the total number of stone procedures.

The best Canadian study to date was performed in 2014 by Ordon et al., utilizing three main data sources: the Ontario Health Insurance Plan (OHIP) database, the Canadian Institute for Health Information Discharge Abstract Database (CIHI-DAD) and the National Ambulatory Care and Reporting System (NACRS) [26]. The authors found that the use of SWL decreased steadily over time with a subsequent increase in ureteroscopy, from 25% in 1991 to 59% in 2010. The authors also found the need for ancillary kidney stone procedures decreased significantly over time, from 23% to 15% in 2010. The authors postulated that while ureteroscopy has seen dramatic technologic advances improving its safety, ease of use, and stone free rates, especially for proximal ureteral stones, minimal technologic advances or corresponding improvements in success with SWL have occurred. Additionally, as access to SWL has remained stable over time, access to URS has improved. Finally, as urologists receive improved training with endoscopic techniques during their residency, increasing comfort level has led to gains in popularity and preference for the procedure.

Matlaga and colleagues were the first to utilize the American Board of Urology case logs to provide a better understanding of current practice patterns of urologists in the United States [21, 27]. The American Board of Urology was started in 1934 to serve as a surgical specialty board for improving standards, promoting competency, and encouraging education in the practice of urology. Urologists may be granted certification by the ABU by completing basic training, thereby demonstrating they have attained a level of knowledge and expertise required for the care of patients with urological diseases. Every urologist certified after 1985 must complete a mandatory recertification every 10 years. A significant portion of the certification is the completion of surgical operative logs describing a 6-consecutive month period prior to application submission. These logs characterize patient demographics including patient age and gender as well as surgeon-specific characteristics including age, certification group, and location of clinical practice. In addition, surgeons report self-appointed sub-specialization in one of five areas (endourology, oncology, pediatrics, andrology, and female urology). Diagnoses are logged according to ICD-9 code and surgical procedures are coded using the CPT code system.

ABU cases logs serve as a unique source of documented clinical practices of urologists in the United States (US) and are a reliable, accurate representation of practice patterns. One of the strengths of the ABU cases logs is its ability to provide important demographic and surgeon characteristics not obtainable from surgical outcomes or administrative databases such as the National Surgical Quality Improvement Project or National Inpatient Sample. Furthermore, case logs represent all urologists in the United States, avoiding referral biases seen in studies completed at academic institutions which may be skewed toward more complex stone cases and recall biases seen in physician surveys. To date, they provide one of the most reliable representations of the workload and practice patterns of urologists in the US.

Matlaga assessed surgical logs from 2004 to 2008 and found that newly trained urologists utilized ureteroscopy in the majority of stone removal procedures (52.0%), whereas urologists in the first and second recertification cohort preferentially utilized shock wave lithotripsy in the majority of their procedures (57.4% and 60.5%, respectively). Definitive explanation of these patterns is not possible from the data set; however, one may formulate several theories from these patterns. It may be that younger urologist approach upper tract stones in fundamentally different ways than their older cohorts. Perhaps younger surgeons who have just completed residency training have more experience and are more comfortable performing endoscopic procedures such as URS and PCNL. On the contrary, Matlaga also postulated that perhaps surgeons who have been in practice have more experience with SWL and are more comfortable performing the procedure. Because SWL was introduced into the clinical stone repertoire in the early 1980s, many of the urologists in the first and second recertification cohorts were trained during this time or may have built their careers on successful SWL treatments.

Building on the work of Matlaga, we reassessed the surgical case logs examining the ten-year period from 2003 to 2012 [28]. We hypothesized that younger urologists would continue to perform URS in numbers that increasingly exceed SWL, as Matlaga and colleagues documented. In addition, we hypothesized that older surgeons would begin to adopt URS in increasing numbers similar to their younger colleagues. Finally, our research focused on the influence of urologic sub specialization. We hypothesized that those surgeons specializing in endourology would perform an increased number of PCNL surgeries relative to non-endourologists. Our data set included a total of 6,620 urologists whom reported case logs over this 10-year period. Based on data from the Cecil G. Sheps Center for Health Services, our study captures a cross section of surgeons representing 70% of the estimated 9,500 urologists practicing in the United States in 2013 [29].

A total of 441,162 total procedures for upper tract urinary calculi were performed: 54.2% ureteroscopy, 41.3% SWL, and 4.5% PCNL. We observed an overall increase in the use of URS from 40.9% in 2003 to 59.6% of all stone procedures in 2012. There was a corresponding drop in use of SWL from 54% to 36.3%. The utilization of PCNL remained stable accounting for 4-5% of all surgeries over this time period. These findings closely mirror the Canadian results of Ordon and colleagues who described a similar rate of ureteroscopic utilization of 59% in 2010.

Because ABU case logs are surgeon-specific, we have the ability to compare experience level, surgeon age, and specialty on stone treatment utilization. New urologists displayed an increase in the use of ureteroscopy, 47.6% to 70.9% over this period (23% increase). More senior surgeons, those undergoing first and second recertification, similarly displayed a rise in use of ureteroscopy from 40% in 2003 to 55% in 2012, a 15% increase. We found that endourologists performed a significantly higher proportion of PCNL than non-endourologists (10.6% vs. 3.69%) and a significantly smaller proportion of SWL (34.2% vs. 42.2%).

The location of clinical practice was examined to assess differences in stone surgery by state and region. We found that the Southeast region logged the highest number of all total stone surgeries in the United States. Yet, when stratified by total population for each US region, there was no statistically significant difference in type of stone surgery performed. When comparing individual states, we found that there are small individual differences among states, but none were found to be statistically significant. Overall, the trend towards the increased use of ureteroscopy and decreased use of SWL was observed in every US geographic region.

Seklehner and colleagues performed a similar analysis of surgical practice patterns in the United States utilizing the 5% Medicare claims data from 2001, 2004, 2007 and 2010 from the Centers for Medicare and Medicaid Services. The Public Use files included multiple datasets encompassing physician and hospital inpatient and outpatient medical claims from a 5% national random sample of beneficiaries [24]. The cohort included a total of 299,920 patients with ureteric stones, and of those 115,200 patients underwent surgery. Interesting, although the Medicare data shows an overall increase by 59% of ureteric calculi prevalence over this 10-year period, the surgical treatment rate remained constant at 38%. They found that men were more likely to undergo treatment for a ureteral stone (OR 1.15, $p<0.001$), whereas ethnic minorities were significantly less likely to be treated (OR=0.84, $p=0.004$). Sekleher's results closely mirror the trend toward ureteroscopy as seen in the ABU case logs data and the Ontario dataset. The predominant surgical approach for ureteral stones was ureteroscopy, leading SWL 65.2% to 33.6%. Only 1.2% of patients underwent ureterolithotomy in the Medicare cohort.

It is clear that the treatment of upper tract calculi continues to evolve and provider specific attributes continue to affect stone treatment. The contemporary literature is in agreement that younger urologists have adopted endoscopic techniques at high frequencies [30]. Interestingly, the newest data available shows that both newly trained urologists and senior-level urologists have adopted endoscopic techniques at such a rapid pace such that all levels of urologists are now performing URS at a higher frequency than SWL. This is in contrast to a number of historical studies which found SWL to be the most commonly performed procedure and the use of URS to predominate only in the junior urologist cohort [21, 30]. Modern ureteroscopic technologies are the products of technologic advances over the last two decades and their development initially favored the adoption by urologists in the initial certification cohort more recently trained in endoscopic techniques. What is interesting is that it appears the adoption of newer technologies has now reached all urologists regardless of length of time in practice.

There are several theories as to why surgeons from all generations are now performing endoscopic procedures at increased frequencies: technologic improvements resulting in decreased costs, surgeon comfort and ease of use, and improvements in surgical outcomes including stone-free and retreatment rates when compared to SWL [31, 32].

As new technologies in surgery become increasingly widespread, such as the dispersion of flexible ureteroscopy over the last 20 years, we see significant improvements in the cost-effectiveness, which may account for its increased use [33]. For example, factors such as improved durability of newer scopes [34], as well as superior efficiency and cost-effectiveness of URS for stones up to and larger than 1 cm when compared with SWL may partially account for these practice pattern changes [35].

Despite the introduction of newer SWL technologies with modifications to improve the efficacy of SWL [36], we observed a decline in SWL use in our study. Is it possible these newer machines have increased potential problems compared to first-generation devices resulting in a decline in their use? Further research is needed to determine if this preference for ureteroscopic techniques is due to SWL inferiority in providing complete treatment of stone burden in a single session. Recent data on newer technologies such as large focus shock wave sources is promising for providing increased efficacy with minimal trauma [36, 37]. An improvement in pulverization and reduction in the number of re-treatments with these newer technologies may lead to a resurgence in use of SWL in the future.

Overall, several studies in our review confirmed that the application of PCNL remained stable and a few studies such as those completed by Ordon and colleagues noticed a decreased in PCNL utilization [26]. Although we have seen technologic advances with improvements in stone fragmentation and decreased complications with PCNL [14, 38, 39], it is likely that PCNL is being reserved for larger or complex stone burdens and its overall increased morbidity may be limiting any expansion in its use. Not surprisingly, these cases are performed in much higher percentages by endourologists who specialize in stone surgery. Our study builds on and confirms similar work by Dr. Jayram and Matlaga of Johns Hopkins University who utilized the database to look specifically at PCNL within the ABU case logs [40]. Younger and fellowship-trained urologists were found to more frequently use PCNL while the majority of senior urologists do not perform this operation. For example, newly certified urologists logged having performed a PCNL in the last six months at a rate of 53% compared with 41% of recertifying urologists and only 29% of those in the second recertification group.

Improved surgical cure and stone-free rates for ureteroscopy compared to SWL might also be driving the change in adoption patterns.[3-7] For example, Wu et al. assessed the treatment of proximal ureteral stones and found a significantly improved stone-free rate following ureteroscopy of 92% vs. 61% when compared to SWL [41]. In addition, a recent study by Scales et al., found that when compared to SWL, ureteroscopy is associated with significantly fewer repeat treatments [42]. These findings confirm previous studies, which demonstrated SWL to have a 20-30% re-treatment rate and associated patient discomfort with passage of fragments [42].

The majority of the studies described in this chapter are not without potential limitations. Because of the observational, prospectively collected nature of most practice patterns study, it is difficult to extrapolate causality to changes in treatment modality usage over time. Several theories have been postulated in this chapter as to why we are seeing these patterns; however, those conclusions cannot be made from the data currently available. Rather, additional studies are needed to better test these hypotheses. The overall accuracy of the most recent practice pattern studies available is strong and to date provides the most reliable representations of the workloads and practice patterns of urologists in the US.

Conclusion

The treatment of upper tract calculi remains an evolving field and provider-specific attributes continue to affect stone treatment decisions. Our research in conjunction with similar studies of modern stone management and practice patterns provides strong evidence that ureteroscopy has surpassed SWL as the primary treatment modality for upper tract stones among both newly trained and senior urologists. PCNL utilization has remained stable over time and continues to be performed in disproportionate numbers by younger urologists and those who specialize in endourology.

As health care spending increases, it is imperative that we identify new ways to improve the value of the care we provide as urologists and understand what factors are influencing treatment modality choices. Surgical practice patterns can be powerful data when accurately captured and have the potential to guide healthcare spending, workforce estimations, and clinical decision-making. Given the current climate of health care, there is no doubt that there exists a pressing need for further illumination of the driving forces behind these trends.

References

[1] Shah J, Whitfield HN. Urolithiasis through the ages. *BJU international.* 2002;89(8):801-10.

[2] Stamatelou KK, Francis ME, Jones CA, Nyberg LM, Curhan GC. Time trends in reported prevalence of kidney stones in the United States: 1976-1994. *Kidney international.* 2003;63(5):1817-23.

[3] Saigal CS, Joyce G, Timilsina AR. Direct and indirect costs of nephrolithiasis in an employed population: opportunity for disease management? *Kidney international.* 2005;68(4):1808-14.

[4] Scales CD, Jr., Smith AC, Hanley JM, Saigal CS. Prevalence of kidney stones in the United States. *European urology.* 2012;62(1):160-5.

[5] Romero V, Akpinar H, Assimos DG. Kidney stones: a global picture of prevalence, incidence, and associated risk factors. *Reviews in urology.* 2010;12(2-3):e86-96.

[6] Scales CD, Jr., Krupski TL, Curtis LH, Matlaga B, Lotan Y, Pearle MS, et al. Practice variation in the surgical management of urinary lithiasis. *J Urol.* 2011;186(1):146-50.

[7] Soucie JM, Thun MJ, Coates RJ, McClellan W, Austin H. Demographic and geographic variability of kidney stones in the United States. *Kidney international.* 1994;46(3):893-9.

[8] Akoudad S, Szklo M, McAdams MA, Fulop T, Anderson CA, Coresh J, et al. Correlates of kidney stone disease differ by race in a multi-ethnic middle-aged population: the ARIC study. *Preventive medicine.* 2010;51(5):416-20.

[9] Hesse A, Brandle E, Wilbert D, Kohrmann KU, Alken P. Study on the prevalence and incidence of urolithiasis in Germany comparing the years 1979 vs. 2000. *European urology.* 2003;44(6):709-13.

[10] Seklehner S, Laudano MA, Jamzadeh A, Del Pizzo JJ, Chughtai B, Lee RK. Trends and inequalities in the surgical management of ureteric calculi in the USA. *BJU international.* 2013.

[11] Albala DM, Assimos DG, Clayman RV, Denstedt JD, Grasso M, Gutierrez-Aceves J, et al. Lower pole I: a prospective randomized trial of extracorporeal shock wave lithotripsy and percutaneous nephrostolithotomy for lower pole nephrolithiasis-initial results. *J Urol.* 2001;166(6):2072-80.

[12] Bagley DH. Expanding role of ureteroscopy and laser lithotripsy for treatment of proximal ureteral and intrarenal calculi. *Current opinion in urology.* 2002;12(4):277-80.

[13] Sammon JD, Ghani KR, Karakiewicz PI, Bhojani N, Ravi P, Sun M, et al. Temporal trends, practice patterns, and treatment outcomes for infected upper urinary tract stones in the United States. *European urology.* 2013;64(1):85-92.

[14] Ghani KR, Sammon JD, Bhojani N, Karakiewicz PI, Sun M, Sukumar S, et al. Trends in percutaneous nephrolithotomy use and outcomes in the United States. *J Urol.* 2013;190(2):558-64.

[15] Pearle MS, Calhoun EA, Curhan GC. Urologic diseases in America project: urolithiasis. *J Urol.* 2005;173(3):848-57.

[16] Preminger GM, Tiselius HG, Assimos DG, Alken P, Buck C, Gallucci M, et al. 2007 guideline for the management of ureteral calculi. *J Urol.* 2007;178(6):2418-34.

[17] Caldwell DM, Ades AE, Higgins JP. Simultaneous comparison of multiple treatments: combining direct and indirect evidence. *Bmj.* 2005;331(7521):897-900.

[18] Matlaga BR, Jansen JP, Meckley LM, Byrne TW, Lingeman JE. Treatment of ureteral and renal stones: a systematic review and meta-analysis of randomized, controlled trials. *J Urol.* 2012;188(1):130-7.

[19] Aboumarzouk OM, Kata SG, Keeley FX, McClinton S, Nabi G. Extracorporeal shock wave lithotripsy (ESWL) versus ureteroscopic management for ureteric calculi. *The Cochrane database of systematic reviews*. 2012;5:Cd006029.

[20] Turney BW, Reynard JM, Noble JG, Keoghane SR. Trends in urological stone disease. *BJU international.* 2012;109(7):1082-7.

[21] Matlaga BR. Contemporary surgical management of upper urinary tract calculi. *J Urol.* 2009;181(5):2152-6.

[22] Bandi G, Best SL, Nakada SY. Current practice patterns in the management of upper urinary tract calculi in the north central United States. *Journal of endourology / Endourological Society.* 2008;22 (4):631-6.

[23] Ghani KR, Sammon JD, Karakiewicz PI, Sun M, Bhojani N, Sukumar S, et al. Trends in surgery for upper urinary tract calculi in the USA using the Nationwide Inpatient Sample: 1999-2009. *BJU international.* 2013;112(2):224-30.

[24] Seklehner S, Laudano MA, Jamzadeh A, Del Pizzo JJ, Chughtai B, Lee RK. Trends and inequalities in the surgical management of ureteric calculi in the USA. *BJU international.* 2014;113(3):476-83.

[25] Lee MC, Bariol SV. Evolution of stone management in Australia. *BJU international.* 2011;108 Suppl 2:29-33.

[26] Ordon M, Urbach D, Mamdani M, Saskin R, D'A Honey RJ, Pace KT. The Surgical Management of Kidney Stone Disease: A Population Based Time Series Analysis. *J Urol.* 2014.

[27] Oberlin DT, Flum A, Bachrach L, Flury SC. PD7-09 Contemporary surgical trends in the managment of upper tract calculi. T*he Journal of Urology.* 2014;191(4, Supplement):e187.

[28] Oberlin DT, Flum AS, Bachrach L, Matulewicz RS, Flury SC. Contemporary Surgical Trends in the Management of Upper Tract Calculi. *J Urol. 2*014.

[29] Raj S. Purthi MEN. Age, gender, and the urology work force: Evolving trends - See more at: *Urology Times*. 2014.

[30] Bird VG, Fallon B, Winfield HN. Practice patterns in the treatment of large renal stones. *Journal of endourology / Endourological Society.* 2003;17(6):355-63.

[31] Preminger GM, Tiselius HG, Assimos DG, Alken P, Buck AC, Gallucci M, et al. 2007 Guideline for the management of ureteral calculi. *European urology.* 2007;52(6):1610-31.

[32] Childs MA, Rangel LJ, Lingeman JE, Krambeck AE. Factors influencing urologist treatment preference in surgical management of stone disease. *Urology*. 2012;79(5):996-1003.
[33] Collins JW, Keeley FX, Jr., Timoney A. Cost analysis of flexible ureterorenoscopy. *BJU international*. 2004;93(7):1023-6.
[34] Traxer O, Dubosq F, Jamali K, Gattegno B, Thibault P. New-generation flexible ureterorenoscopes are more durable than previous ones. *Urology*. 2006;68(2):276-9; discussion 80-1.
[35] Parker BD, Frederick RW, Reilly TP, Lowry PS, Bird ET. Efficiency and cost of treating proximal ureteral stones: Shock wave lithotripsy versus ureteroscopy plus holmium:yttrium-aluminum-garnet laser. *Urology*. 2004;64(6):1102-6.
[36] Bhojani N, Lingeman JE. Shockwave lithotripsy-new concepts and optimizing treatment parameters. *The Urologic clinics of North America*. 2013;40(1):59-66.
[37] Rassweiler JJ, Knoll T, Kohrmann KU, McAteer JA, Lingeman JE, Cleveland RO, et al. Shock wave technology and application: an update. *European urology*. 2011;59(5):784-96.
[38] Preminger GM. Percutaneous nephrolithotomy: an extreme technical makeover for an old technique. Archivio italiano di urologia, andrologia: organo ufficiale [di] Societa italiana di ecografia urologica e nefrologica/ Associazione ricerche in urologia. 2010;82(1):23-5.
[39] Lehman DS, Hruby GW, Phillips C, Venkatesh R, Best S, Monga M, et al. Prospective randomized comparison of a combined ultrasonic and pneumatic lithotrite with a standard ultrasonic lithotrite for percutaneous nephrolithotomy. *Journal of endourology / Endourological Society*. 2008;22(2):285-9.
[40] Jayram G, Matlaga BR. Contemporary Practice Patterns Associated with Percutaneous Nephrolithotomy Among Certifying Urologists. *Journal of endourology / Endourological Society*. 2014.
[41] Wu CF, Shee JJ, Lin WY, Lin CL, Chen CS. Comparison between extracorporeal shock wave lithotripsy and semirigid ureterorenoscope with holmium:YAG laser lithotripsy for treating large proximal ureteral stones. *J Urol*. 2004;172(5 Pt 1):1899-902.
[42] Scales CD, Jr, Lai JC, Dick AW, et al. COmparative effectiveness of shock wave lithotripsy and ureteroscopy for treating patients with kidney stones. *JAMA Surgery*. 2014.

In: Urolithiasis
Editor: Joseph Fletcher
ISBN: 978-1-63463-500-4

Chapter 3

Emergency Shockwave Lithotripsy: Past, Present and Future

Andreas Bourdoumis*[1], *MD, FEBU, FES* and *Theodora Stasinou*[2], *MD, MRCS
[1]Locum Consultant Urological Surgeon,
Royal Devon and Exeter NHS Foundation Trust
[2]Core Surgical Trainee, Royal Devon and Exeter NHS Foundation Trust,
Exeter, UK

Abstract

With growing socioeconomic pressure on the health systems worldwide, there is an ever growing need for efficient delivery of care with the best possible results and minimal complications. In the field of Urology and stone disease in particular, shockwave lithotripsy has revolutionized the way lithiasis is managed. The latest development involves the delivery of shockwaves into the acutely obstructing ureteric stone in the form of emergency lithotripsy (eSWL). It allows for rapid pain relief and stone expulsion, thereby reducing morbidity, operating lists waiting times and time off work.

In this chapter, we shall describe the principles of shockwave lithotripsy in brief, as well as the indications and contraindications, as a prelude to the more specialized circumstances of emergency lithotripsy. We shall outline the basic pathophysiologic principles behind emergency treatment and the evidence behind the evolution of a dedicated protocol that produces excellent results in the context of day case treatment.

We shall also describe a referral pathway specifically designed to funnel patients into the service within a specified time frame suitable for the application of emergency shockwave treatment.

Introduction

With growing socioeconomic pressure on the health systems worldwide, there is an ever growing need for efficient delivery of care with the best possible results and minimal complications. In the field of Urology and stone disease in particular, shockwave lithotripsy has revolutionized the way lithiasis is managed.

In this chapter, we shall describe the principles of shockwave lithotripsy in brief, as well as the indications and contraindications, as a prelude to the more specialized circumstances of emergency lithotripsy. We shall outline the basic pathophysiologic principles behind emergency treatment and the evidence behind the evolution of a dedicated protocol that produces excellent results in the context of day case treatment.

The Evolution of Shockwave Lithotripsy - General Principles

Since its first scientific and clinical descriptions by Chaussy in the early 80s, extracorporeal shockwave lithotripsy (ESWL) has truly revolutionized the urologic management of stone disease and remains the only noninvasive surgical treatment modality for urinary tract calculi. [1-3] With expanding use and gain of clinical experience, SWL was added to the endourologic armamentarium of stone treatment. Since the first HM-1 (Human Model-1) machine developed by Dornier and its subsequent modifications (HM-2 and HM-3), several lithotripters have been developed over the years, reaching the era of forth generation lithotripters at present. The basic physic properties underlining the function of stone disintegration involve the generation of an acoustic sound wave by a power source (focal point 1) that will be accurately delivered to the point of interest (focal point 2) i.e., the stone. Acoustic sound waves have nonlinear pressure characteristics and are non-harmonic, in contrast to ultrasonic sound waves. There are two principle types of shock wave generators. The supersonic amplitude emitters transform electrical current energy from a spark gap electrode into a shock wave by releasing that energy in a confined space under water. A rapidly expanding gas bubble is formed as a result of water vaporization around the tip of the electrode. This bubble then collapses and the resulting shock wave is reflected towards the target by a metal hemi-ellipsoid surface. This is the electrohydraulic principle of shockwave lithotripsy and was utilized in the original Dornier machines. The finite amplitude emitters produce shock waves as a result of displacement of material surfaces when electrical current is applied across them. In the electromagnetic type of emitter, two cylindrical plates separated by a thin insulator are electrically charged to create a local magnetic field. The plates are thus displaced and upon their collapse a shock wave is generated that is focused with the aid of a concave acoustic lens. In the piezoelectric type of emitter, an electrical discharge causes a ceramic component to elongate in such a manner that the surface is displaced and an acoustic pulse is generated. Thousands of such components are placed on the concave side of a spheric surface and the pulse is directed toward the focal point in high stress, strain, and cavitation pressures (Table 1). Shock waves result in fragmentation as a result of focused energy transmission to the target, where they cause erosion and shattering. Cavitational forces result in erosion at the entry and exit sites of the shock wave. Shattering results from energy absorption with stress, strain, and shear forces (Figure 1). [4]

The latest developments in lithotripter machines are the product of modification and improvements along the lines of the fundamental physical properties of their predecessors. The size of the effective focal zone is frequently the focus of modification, in order to achieve optimal pressure and energy distribution (Table 2). Multifunctional machines were created, that have either a modular design, where all components are separate and may be assembled according to need, or an integrated design where all components are integrated in the machine and adapted to their function. A third design (hybrid) offers integration of imaging and therapy head in a common console with a detached treatment table. One of the latest innovations has been the development of dual shockwave generator lithotroptors. Such are the Twinheads Th-101 ® and the Duet Magna ® models. The Twinheads (TH) 101 lithotripter (FMD, Lorton, Virginia, USA) is an electro hydraulic integrated system using two sources perpendicular to each other that deliver a synchronous twin pulse. An initial study by Sheir et al., has proven safety and efficacy of the method. [5] In a subsequent prospective randomized trial comparing it to the Dornier S® (Dornier MedTech Europe, Germany) lithotripter, the Twinheads® model presented significant clinical advantages in stone free rates, degree of renal impairment and tissue injury. [6] The Duet Magna ® model from Direx is an integrated lithotripter produced in electro hydraulic and electromagnetic versions that provides two independent generator/reflector systems at 72 degree angle to each other, attempting thus to minimize treatment duration. With the availability of two shock wave sources focused on a single target, the operator has the option to choose the shock wave source location or dual source operation. This combination of two oblong focal points creates the unique 'butterfly'' focal area. Localization is possible with fluoroscopy and ultrasound and the system is operated via a digital console with broad image analysis and positioning capabilities. Handa et al., have tested the Duet ® in porcine kidneys and found the degree of renal impairment to be comparable to, but more variable than that observed with a conventional electrohydraulic lithotripter both in synchronous and alternating modes. [7, 8] Clinical studies in humans have produced a stone free rate of 83-85% without significant complications. [9, 10] The procedure was performed under intravenous sedation in the majority of patients. Further clinical studies are required to establish analgesia requirements for effective fragmentation with minimal discomfort. The Storz Modulith SLX-F2 (Karl Storz, Tubingen, Germany) represents the latest evolution in integrated electromagnetic shockwave generators. The aperture of the therapy head with a diameter of 300 mm provides an area of approximately 700 cm^2 for coupling. As a result, the energy density can be kept at a very low level at the patient skin and minimize analgesia requirements. This modern unit is also equipped with touch screen controls and state-of-the-art software systems, such as the LithoPos® (automatic stone positioning system) and the StorM-Base® (patient and treatment parameter storage and evaluation), as well as the DICOM® module for long-term archiving. The combination of integrated ultrasound targeting enables the SLX-F2 to serve as a complete endourologic suite for a variety of minimally invasive procedures. The efficacy of the electromagnetic generators is well demonstrated. [11] In a series from a single center with single operator experience with two types of lithotripter (electrohydraulic and electromagnetic) both were found to be equally efficacious, with similar safety profiles. [12] The Wolf Piezolith 3000 is an example of a modular design, piezoelectric machine. It may incorporate both fluoroscopic and inline ultrasonographic real-time monitoring of lithotripsy and provide further uses in conjunction with the multifunctional treatment table. Patient positioning is automatic software assisted with in-picture navigation. The piezoelectric element produces a penetration depth of 165mm, while the direct focusing ability of the piezoelectric shockwaves can be adapted to the individual indication and minimize patient discomfort.

Table 1. Characteristics of the first widely used commercial lithotripter models

Company	Machine	Water coupling	Energy source	Analgesia	Imaging modality
Dornier	HM3/HM4 ®	Wet (Bath tub) / Dry (Bag)	Electrohydraulic	General/Epidural	Fluoroscopy
Technomed	1050 ®	Wet (Basin)	Electrohydraulic	General/Epidural	Ultrasound
Siemens	Lithostar ®	Dry (Tube)	Electromagnetic	General/Epidural/Analgesia	Fluoroscopy
EDAP	LT-01 ®	Dry (Bag)	Piezoelectric	Analgesia	Ultrasound
Richard Wolf	Piezolith 2200 ®	Wet(pool)	Piezoelectric	Analgesia	Ultrasound

Table 2. Comparative aspects of the three main shockwave modalities with respective focal areas and functional characteristics

	electrohydraulic	electromagnetic	piezoelectric
	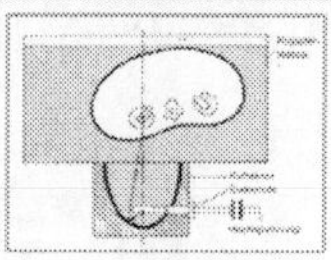	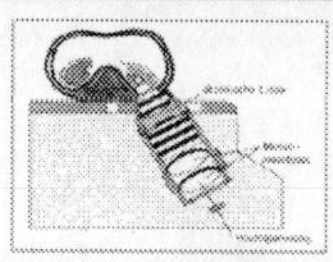	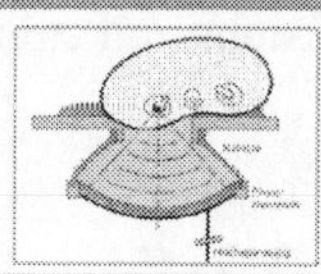
Focal geometry	20 mm / 12 mm	40 mm / 8 mm	20 mm / 3 mm
Energy	+++	++(+)	+
Efficacy	+++	++(+)	+(+)
Precision	+	+++	+++
Pain	+++	++	+
Arrhythmia	+++	+	+
Costs	++	+	+

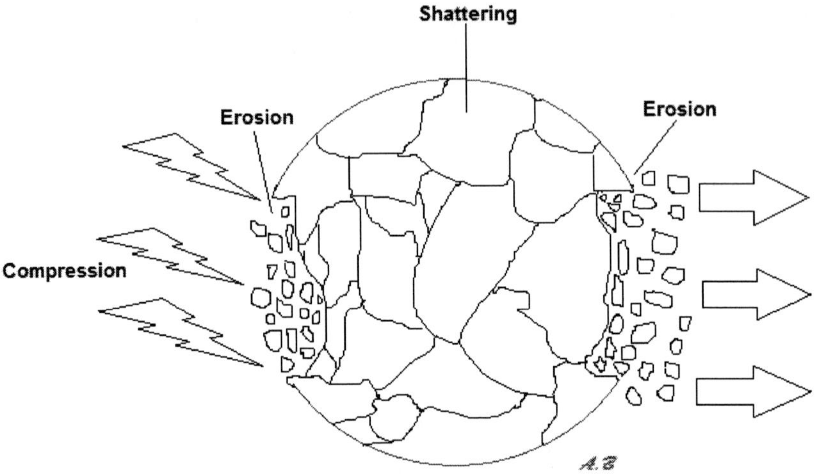

Figure 1. Schematic representation of the various forces and resulting effect of shockwave application to a urinary tract stone.

The control unit consists of a wide touch screen panel with multiple controls and remote operation also possible. The model is also available as a mobile unit that may be transported across sites. In a comparative study with the Storz lithotripter, Albino and Marucco found the two machines to be comparable with regards to number of shock waves per session, the number of sessions and stone free rates (93% vs. 91% respectively). [13]

Contemporary Lithotripsy by Shockwave - The Concept of Emergency Treatment

International urologic associations of considerable repute (EAU, AUA, SIU) have regularly issue and update guidelines for effective management of renal and ureteral stones. As a general cut-off, a size of 2 cm in the kidney is considered the upper limit for SWL, whereas in the ureter, several studies have reported poor stone free rates for stones larger than 1 cm. [14-16] In their recent meta-analysis, Matlaga et al., conclude in favor of ureteroscopy for the management of distal ureteric stones, whereas for proximal and renal stones no definite conclusion could be deducted due to heterogeneity among the studies that was so great as to preclude any meaningful comparison. [17] Acute colic due to obstruction by a ureteric stone can be managed expectantly in the first instance, as spontaneous elimination may occur in 16-98% of cases according to the literature that is usually supplemented with analgesics, most commonly no-steroid anti-inflammatory medication (NSAIDs). [18, 19] The combination of a NSAID with a-blockers has been shown to improve spontaneous stone passage; following numerous studies, medical expulsive treatment is now an establish means of acute stone management. [20] Nevertheless, due to the wide variation of spontaneous stone elimination, additional treatment is often required. The choice of further intervention is largely dependent on stone size and location, as demonstrated by numerous early studies that compared between extracorporeal shock wave lithotripsy (SWL) and ureteroscopy (URS). [21-24] Furthermore, in the latest Cochrane review comparing ureteroscopy and shockwave lithotripsy for ureteric stones, Aboumarzouk et al., conclude that ureteroscopic removal of ureteral stones achieves a greater stone-free state, but with a higher complication rate and longer hospital stay. [25]

The concept of emergency shockwave lithotripsy in the management of acute ureteral colic caused by an obstructing ureteric stone started to develop in the early 90s, when Cass et al., first coined the term 'in situ' SWL. [26] They described treating ureteric stones within 14 days of presentation and producing stone free rates between 78-93% for partial and complete obstruction, respectively, at 3 months follow up. In the same decade, Doublet et al., published their results of 67 patients who received in situ shockwave lithotripsy with a piezo-electric machine for acute colic and presented an overall one month stone-free rate of 94%. [27] Later, Tligui et al., reported a stone free rate of 82% at three months follow up in a study of 200 patients and a mean stone size of 7 mm, again with the use of a piezo-electric shockwave generator. [28] In a subsequent trial enrolling 100 patients, Tombal et al., randomized to medical therapy alone or combined with lithotripsy within 6 hours of pain onset and described an increase in SFR by 13% for proximal ureteric stones (mean size: 5 mm) within 48 hours of treatment. Patients were treated by use of an electromagnetic shockwave generator and standard analgesia. [29]

Owing to the wide variety of makes and models of lithotripters, with different generators and energies, and subtle variations in overall patient care among investigators, it becomes difficult to make comparisons between series of reported data. For example, for a given stone-free rate, one machine may require multiple re-treatments or subsequent stent placements. Denstedt and colleagues described the use of an "efficiency quotient" to take such factors into account as follows:

Efficiency Quotient (EQ) = % Stone-free Divided by
(100 + % Re-Treated + % Auxiliary Procedures) [30]

In their prospective study, Kravchick et al., examined the correlation of stone location (i.e. upper ureter) with success. The stone-free rates were 72% and 64% in the study and control groups respectively. Of note, they also presented their results by use of the efficiency quotient, which were 53% and 44% for the respective groups, albeit in a small total number of patients (n=53). [31] In another prospective study by Kumar et al., one hundred and sixty consecutive patients with a single radiopaque upper ureteral stone of less than 10 mm were randomized to early (< 48 hours) versus late (> 48 hours) SWL using an electromagnetic lithotripter. The authors reported stone free rates at three months of 86.3% vs. 76.2%, respectively, without demonstration of statistically significant difference (p=0.34). The modified EQ was 67.2% vs. 59.4% respectively. [32] In our initial series of emergency SWL for ureteric stones using the Modulith® SLX-F2, the stone free rate 73.2%. [33] In subsequent analysis of a larger cohort of patients, the stone free rate was 86.9% (unpublished data). In our unpublished data, the efficiency quotient was 73% for the emergency treatment group, which is the highest published to date, according to our knowledge. In both studies, stone size and Hounsfield unit (HU) attenuation value on non-contrast CT were consistently found to be predictors of successful outcome, i.e., stone disintegration with two sessions of shockwave treatment delivered in a standardized manner. Earlier studies showed a disintegration rate of 85% with the Modulith SL 20. [34] Tiselius et al., reported stone-free rates over 97% for ureteric stones using the classic and F2 machines. [35] However, in the most recent randomized controlled trial by Zehnder et al., comparing the HM3 to the Modulith® SLX-F2 SWL device confirmed that the older HM3 device has better outcomes. [36]

The results from the current studies substantiate a cut-off size of 8 mm and attenuation value of less than 900 HU in computed tomography as predictors for successful lithotripsy in the acute setting. Similar cut-off attenuation values have been previously described in the literature. [37, 38] We believe these results are adequately explained by the cascade of events common to all types of stone in the urinary tract. A patient undergoing elective SWL is subject to more waiting time compared to a patient on emergency SWL. Hence the stones treated on the elective list will eventually be bigger, and as a result additional sessions would be required more frequently. This could explain both the finding of a bigger mean stone size and the need for a second SWL more frequently in the elective group. In addition, it is possible that adjuvant crystallization occurs at the same time, producing harder stones, shown by the greater attenuation of the stones in the elective treatment group. Furthermore to existing evidence, the time to luminal edema seems to play a critical part to stone impaction and subsequent outcome, either by SWL or ureteroscopy. [39-41] By treating stones within a 72-hour window, there is a chance of creating smaller fragments that would eventually pass with greater ease, even with the additional obstruction caused by tissue swelling.

If a definition was to be formulated for emergency SWL, that could be that it represents treatment by extracorporeal shockwaves with intent to break an acutely obstructing, radiopaque ureteric stone within 72 hours of presentation of symptoms in a non infected system and in the absence of absolute contraindications for SWL. Indeed, this definition encompasses all the prerequisites for emergency extracorporeal lithotripsy. An impacted stone creates ureteral edema gradually over 24–72 h, impairing stone clearance by preventing the formation of the chamber–liquid interface. Once established, further movement of the stone is prohibited and pain resolves only when sufficient time has passed and the ureter accommodates the calculus by dilation, so that it no longer obstructs completely but only partially and intermittently. An attempt to completely fragment the stone within that time frame maximizes the chances for spontaneous stone passage, thereby reducing analgesic requirement and saving time of work.

Indications and Limitations

Suitable candidates for urgent SWL include those who present within 72 hrs of pain caused by a radiopaque ureteric calculus in a non-infected system. Apart from these indications, all the absolute and relative contraindications that pertain for conventional lithotripsy apply for urgent treatment as well. Uncorrected coagulopathy and/or active anticoagulation, active urinary tract infection and pregnancy constitute absolute contraindications, whereas arterial aneurysm in the vicinity, musculoskeletal deformities, the presence of cardiac pacemaker and/or implanted defibrillator and obesity are relative contraindications, as treatment may go forward in carefully selected individuals by carefully considering effectiveness of treatment and benefit versus risk. For example, patients with a pacemaker can be treated with SWL, provided that appropriate technical precautions are taken. These include adjustment of the pacemaker by a qualified technician prior to treatment in an electromagnetic lithotripter. [42] Patients with implanted cardioverter defibrillators must be managed with reprogramming of the firing mode temporarily during SWL treatment. [42] However, this might not be always necessary with new-generation lithotripters and the specific manufacturer recommendations should always be sought for and taken into consideration. Pregnancy is a contraindication due to the unpredictable consequences of the transmitted shockwave energy to the fetus. [43]

Primary ureteroscopy appears to be a safe and more effective alternative to SWL for dealing with ureteric stones in pregnancy. [44]

It is obvious that adherence to the above recommendations contributes towards safe delivery of care and successful lithotripsy. Further improvements that contribute towards the same goal are described in the following section

The Future of Emergency Shockwave Lithotripsy - Technology and Management

Technology

Advances in technology contribute to a great extent in developing new treatment strategies. Extracorporeal SWL revolutionized the treatment of urolithiasis. Until recently, the progress in lithotripter technology focused mainly on the integration of the shock wave source into multifunctional fluoroscopic tables, rather than improving the efficacy of energy delivery. Promising new data regarding increased efficacy and minimal trauma of SW sources with large focus aim at improving the actual stone free rate per session. It is interesting that even after 30 years of intensive research, the ideal device has yet to be presented. That device should be highly efficient in stone disintegration with minor, if any, associated side effects and few required sessions. However, there are additional considerations, such as performing the treatment with minimal analgesic requirements. Larger aperture systems enable treatment almost without anesthesia; however, such systems have a very small focal zone requiring multiple sessions. New theories for stone disintegration favor the use of shock wave sources with larger focal zones. Use of slower pulse rates, ramping strategies, and adequate coupling of the shock wave head can significantly increase the efficacy and safety of SWL. Indeed, some of the large focus lithotripters already enable SWL without any anesthesia or analgesia. However, these energy sources have to be combined with sophisticated localization systems. Early trials with charge-coupled device (CCD) ultrasound indicate that the duplex signal may show when the stone is adequately hit by the shock wave and, probably also, when the stone starts to fragment. [45]

The *electroconductive system (*EDAP-TMS, Lyon, France) employs electrodes in a highly conductive solution, resulting in repeatable spark location due to shorter and self-adjusting inter-electrode distance to compensate for electrode wear. [46] Electrode lifetime exceeds 40,000 impulses. *Electromagnetic* and *piezoelectric* sources provide stable shock wave release lasting for >1 million shocks; however, instability of acoustic output may occur. [47] *Adaptation of the focal zone to stone size and localization* seems to be another reasonable innovation. Some manufacturers have found ways to adjust focal width to suit such clinical applications. In the Modulith SLX-F2 (Storz Medical, Germany), two focal sizes are obtained by modifying pulse duration using the same electromagnetic source. The larger focal zone (50 × 9 mm) is recommended for renal stones and the smaller focus (28 × 6 mm) for ureteral stones. However, there is no clinical study that analyzes the impact of the concept. De Sio et al. [48] evaluated only the smaller (original) focus size, and in the comparative study from Berne et al. [49] only the larger focus was taken. In this randomized controlled trial, the 3-month stone-free rate of HM3 was slightly higher compared to the use of F2 focus of the Modulith (90% vs. 81%). However, there are no data when using the standard smaller focus. *Double-layer arrangement of piezoelectric elements* in Piezolith 3000 (Richard Wolf GmbH) increased shock wave energy after reducing the aperture from 50 to 30 cm. [50] Modifying the synchronization of both traveling waves allows variation of delay and pulse formation, resulting in three focal zones. However, the treatment requires intravenous analgesia and resulting stone free rates are low (64%). [51, 52] *Broad-focus, low-pressure lithotripters* (LithoSpace, LithoGold 380, Xinin XX-ES) have recently become the focus of attention as it appears that focal width affects stone disintegration in several ways. [46, 53] Early clinical results show that treatment is possible without any anesthesia and with minimal renal trauma.

Management Strategies

The concept of urgent or emergency lithotripsy represents the latest development in management. It allows for rapid pain relief and stone expulsion, thereby reducing morbidity, operating lists waiting times and time off work. In order to obtain the maximum out of the available technology, treatments must be carefully tailored to individual needs based on best practice, evidence-based guidelines.

Suitable candidates should be directed by a safe and time-efficient referral pathway to tertiary care centers with the appropriate facilities and experience. At the Royal London Hospital, Barts Health NHS Trust, London, UK, a pathway was developed during the period 2012-2013 that allows timely referral of patients suffering from ureteric colic within 72 hours of presentation to an allocated slot on the daily lithotripter treatment schedule. Following careful design and advertising of the service, physicians from East London can now fill in a referral proforma and e –mail their request into a secure address with encrypted access, available only to the SWL operator, which is a dedicated medical professional in the case of our institution. Upon review of request to ensure appropriateness, the operator notifies the respective administrative services again with electronic correspondence in order to request inclusion into the especially allocated treatment slot for urgent SWL on the daily schedule. In this way, personal data and information are protected; patients are treated within the specified time window and with respect to indication, while the maximum of resources is put to good use. Other than basic demographic data, the proforma includes questions on time and nature of presentation, presence or absence of urinary tract infection verified by urinalysis, presence of ureteric calculus on non-contrast abdominal CT which is visible on the plain XR scout film, past medical and surgical history, medication history, as well as any previous history of stone formation and spontaneous stone passage. As a standard, the pathway offers two (2) sessions of SWL, the second within 2 weeks, following which the patient is assessed with new imaging, preferably a low dose CT and symptoms. If satisfactory clearance is achieved, the individual is further referred for metabolic stone analysis and consultation on stone prevention. In case of residual stone and/or symptoms, the patient is scheduled for active removal of the remaining stones by ureteroscopy and laser fragmentation. According to the particular circumstances, a ureteric stent may be inserted prior to definite treatment.

Standardization of treatment technique and stone physical properties is equally important. There is now sufficient evidence in the literature to support a systematic and standard approach to lithotripsy. Based on results from other emergency SWL series as well as our own, we propose a cut-off size of 8 mm and attenuation value of 900 HU in order to perform emergency SWL on ureteric stones with reasonable chances of success. Shockwave delivery parameters are also standardised. At our institution, we treat urgent cases with frequency ranging between 60-90 shocks per minute, as we consider this to be the optimal range in the acute and elective setting. Lee et al. in 2011 propose SWL treatment at a frequency of 60 shocks/min yielded better outcomes, such as a lower number of SWL sessions, and had an increased success rate compared with SWL at 120 shocks/min. [54] Mazzucchi et al. found no significant differences in the stone-free and complication rates were observed by reducing the total number of impulses from 4000 to 3000 and the frequency from 90 to 60 impulses per minute. [55] Chacko et al. favors a frequency reduction, arguing that 90 sw/min treatment gave better results in terms of stone fragmentation compared to 120 sw/min. [56] Total number of shockwaves delivered do not exceed 4000, as per manufacturer recommendations, while energy is increased in a step wise manner to reach the maximum level allowed for the ureter by the manufacturer (8 Joules). In animal models, stepwise power increases (18–20–22 kV) during treatment gave better results in terms of stone comminuting compared with power decreases or leveling (96.5% vs. 89% vs. 87.6%, respectively). [57] An absolute prerequisite is comfortable and relatively pain-free experience by the patient throughout the session. We provide standard analgesia in the form of a non-steroidal anti-inflammatory per rectum 5-10 minutes before the procedure, with respect to allergy and side effect profile. Treatment is discontinued in case of intolerance or increasing pain. Patients should be prescribed medical expulsive treatment, as it has been proven to expedite fragment expulsion and increase stone free rates, as well as reduce additional analgesic requirements. [58, 59]

Efforts to integrate all available knowledge into predicting success are ongoing. Nomograms were introduced by Kanao et al. correlating stone size, location, and numbers to predict stone-free rates after the procedure using a Dornier Lithotripter D. [60] Recently, Nakajiima and Kanao validated the nomograms, finding a remarkable area under the curve (AUC) value of 0.725. [61] This remarkable effort to predict outcome was until now limited to the Dornier machine. Vakalopoulos avoided this gap by developing a mathematical model to predict extracorporeal shockwave lithotripsy outcomes where predictive equations can be created for different lithotripters. [62] Wiesenthal JD et al. developed a comprehensive nomogram to predict renal and ureteral stone shock wave lithotripsy outcomes, dependent on patient and stone related factors. These factors included stone location, were age, body mass index, stone size, mean stone density ($p < 0.01$) and skin to stone distance. [63]

Conclusion

Emergency SWL is an effective, non-invasive method for treating acutely obstructing ureteral stones. Stone size, stone attenuation measured in Hounsfield units and treatment within 72 hours seem to be the main predictive factors the influence outcome and need for re-treatment. There is sufficient evidence to offer this option in the acute setting for the respective group of patients. With continuous technological improvement and enhancement of clinical experience, more patients with renal colic are likely to enjoy a pain and stone free status earlier and with lesser requirement for additional therapy and intervention.

References

[1] Eisenberger F, Chaussy C. Contact-free renal stone fragmentation with shock waves. *Urol Res* 1978; 6: 111.

[2] Chaussy C, Brende, W, Schmiedt E. Extracorporeally induced destruction of kidney stones by shock waves. *Lancet* 1980; 2: 1265.

[3] Chaussy C, Schmiedt E, Jocham D, et al. First clinical experience with extracorporeally induced destruction of kidney stones by shock waves. *J Urol* 1982; 127: 417.

[4] Pfister RC, Papanicolaou N, Yoder IC. Urinary extracorporeal shock wave lithotripsy: equipment, techniques, and overview. *Urol Radiol.* 1988;10(1):39-45.

[5] Sheir KZ, El-Diasty TA, Ismail AM. Evaluation of a synchronous twin-pulse technique for shock wave lithotripsy: the first prospective clinical study. *BJU Int.* 2005;95(3):389-93.

[6] Sheir KZ, Elhalwagy SM, Abo-Elghar ME, Ismail AM, Elsawy E, El-Diasty TA, et al. Evaluation of a synchronous twin-pulse technique for shock wave lithotripsy: a prospective randomized study of effectiveness and safety in comparison to standard single-pulse technique. *BJU Int.* 2008;101(11):1420-6.

[7] Handa RK, McAteer JA, Willis LR, Pishchalnikov YA, Connors BA, Ying J, et al. Dual-head lithotripsy in synchronous mode: acute effect on renal function and morphology in the pig. *BJU Int.* 2007;99(5):1134-42.

[8] Handa RK, McAteer JA, Evan AP, Connors BA, Pishchalnikov YA, Gao S. Assessment of renal injury with a clinical dual head lithotriptor delivering 240 shock waves per minute. *J Urol.* 2009;181(2):884-9.

[9] Varea S, Santomil F, Penida A, Grillo C, Quezada J. *Electromagnetic Double Shockwave Lithotripsy: Initial experience.* Abstract-Presentation at CAU Chilie 2010.

[10] Abbaraju J, Anjum A, Sahai S, Madaan S, Marsh H, Sriprasad S. *Initial experience with a new dual shockwave lithotripter in the management of upper urinary tract calculi.* Abstract- Presentation at EAU 2010.

[11] Sheir KZ, Madbouly K, Elsobky E. Prospective randomized comparative study of the effectiveness and safety of electrohydraulic and electromagnetic extracorporeal shock wave lithotriptors. *J Urol.* 2003;170(2 Pt 1):389-92.

[12] Jamshaid A, Ather MH, Hussain G, Khawaja KB. Single center, single operator comparative study of the effectiveness of electrohydraulic and electromagnetic lithotripters in the management of 10- to 20-mm single upper urinary tract calculi. *Urology.* 2008; 72(5):991-5.

[13] Albino G, Marucco EC. Comparison of ESWL outcome between Wolf Piezolith 3000 vs. storz Modulith Slk. it is the man who makes efficient the machine. *Arch Ital Urol Androl.* 2012;84(4):268-71.

[14] Turk C, Knoll T, Petrik A, Sarica K, Skolarikos A, Straub M, Seitz C; members of the European Association of Urology (EAU) Guidelines Office. Guidelines on Urolithiasis. In: *EAU Guidelines,* edition presented at the 28th EAU Annual Congress, Milan 2013.

[15] Albala DM, Assimos DG, Clayman RV, Denstedt JD, Grasso M, Gutierrez-Aceves J, Kahn RI, et al. Lower pole I: a prospective randomized trial of extracorporeal shock wave lithotripsy and percutaneous nephrostolithotomy for lower pole nephrolithiasis-initial results. *J Urol.* 2001;166(6):2072-80.

[16] Pearle MS, Lingeman JE, Leveillee R, Kuo R, Preminger GM, Nadler RB, Macaluso J, et al. Prospective randomized trial comparing shock wave lithotripsy and ureteroscopy for lower pole caliceal calculi 1 cm or less. *J Urol.* 2008;179(5 Suppl):S69-73.

[17] Matlaga BR, Jansen JP, Meckley LM, Byrne TW, Lingeman JE. Treatment of ureteral and renal stones: a systematic review and meta-analysis of randomized, controlled trials. *J Urol.* 2012;188(1):130-7.

[18] Skolarikos A, Laguna MP, Alivizatos G, Kural AR, de la Rosette JJ. The role for active monitoring in urinary stones: a systematic review. *J Endourol.* 2010 ;24(6):923-30.

[19] Morse RM, Resnick IM. Ureteral calculi: natural history and treatment in an era of advanced technology. *J Urol* 1991;145:263–5.

[20] Seitz C, Liatsikos E, Porpiglia F, et al. Medical Therapy to Facilitate the Passage of Stones: What Is the Evidence? *Eur Urol* 2009 Sep;56(3):455-71.

[21] Anderson KR, Keetch DW, Albala DM, Chandhoke PS, McClennan BL, Clayman RV. Optimal therapy for the ureteral stone: extracorporeal shockwave lithotripsy versus ureteroscopy. *J Urol* 1994;152:62–5.

[22] Deliveliotis C, Stavropoulos NI, Koutsokoulis G, Kostakopoulos A, Dimopoulos C. Distal ureteral calculi: ureteroscopy vs ESWL. A prospective analysis. *Int Urol* Nephrol 1996;28:627–31.

[23] Clayman RV. Outpatient treatment of middle and lower ureteric stones: extra-corporeal shock wave lithotripsy versus ureteroscopic laser lithotripsy. *J Urol* 1999;162:1876–7.

[24] Turk MT, Jenkins AD. A comparison of ureteroscopy to in situ extracorporeal shock wave lithotripsy for the treatment of distal ureteral calculi. *J Urol* 1999;161: 45–7.

[25] Aboumarzouk OM, Kata SG, Keeley FX, McClinton S, Nabi G. Extracorporeal shock wave lithotripsy (ESWL) versus ureteroscopic management for ureteric calculi. *Cochrane Database Syst Rev.* 2012; 16;5:CD006029

[26] Cass AS. In situ extracorporeal shock wave lithotripsy for obstructing ureteral stones with acute renal colic. *J Urol.* 1992; 148(6):1786-7.

[27] Doublet JD, Tchala K, Tligui M, Ciofu C, Gattegno B, Thibault P. In situ extracorporeal shock wave lithotripsy for acute renal colic due to obstructing ureteral stones. *Scand J Urol Nephrol.* 1997; 31 (2):137-9.

[28] Tligui M, El Khadime MR, Tchala K, Haab F, Traxer O, Gattegno B, Thibault P. Emergency extracorporeal shock wave lithotripsy (ESWL) for obstructing ureteral stones. *Eur Urol,* 2003; 43(5):552-5.

[29] Tombal B, Mawlawi H, Feyaerts A, Wese FX, Opsomer R, Van Cangh PJ. Prospective randomized evaluation of emergency extracorporeal shock wave lithotripsy (ESWL) on the short-time outcome of symptomatic ureteral stones. *Eur Urol,* 2005; 47(6):855-9.

[30] Denstedt J, Clayman RV, Preminger GM. Efficiency quotient as a means of comparing lithotripters. *J Endourol* 1990; 4: 100.

[31] Kravchick S, Bunkin I, Stepnov E, Peled R, Agulansky L, Cytron S. Emergency extracorporeal shockwave lithotripsy for acute renal colic caused by upper urinary-tract stones. *J Endourol,* 2005;19(1):1-4.

[32] Kumar A, Mohanty NK, Jain M, Prakash S, Arora RP. A prospective randomized comparison between early (<48 hours of onset of colicky pain) versus delayed shockwave lithotripsy for symptomatic upper ureteral calculi: a single center experience. *J Endourol.* 2010; 24(12):2059-66.

[33] Panah A, Patel S, Bourdoumis A, Kachrilas S, Buchholz N, Masood J. Factors predicting success of emergency extracorporeal shockwave lithotripsy (eESWL) in ureteric calculi--a single centre experience from the United Kingdom (UK). *Urolithiasis.* 2013;41(5):437-41.

[34] Rassweiler J, Henkel TO, Joyce AD, Köhrmann KU, Manning M, Alken P. Extracorporeal shock wave lithotripsy of ureteric stones with the Modulith SL20. *Br J Urol.* 1992;70:594–9.

[35] Tiselius HG. How efficient is extracorporeal shockwave lithotripsy with modern lithotripters for removal of ureteral stones. *J Endourol.* 2008;22:249–55.

[36] Zehnder P, Roth B, Birkhäuser F, Schneider S, Schmutz R, Thalmann GN, Studer UE. A prospective randomised trial comparing the modified HM3 with the MODULITH® SLX-F2 lithotripter. *Eur Urol.* 2011; 59(4):637-44.

[37] Perks AE, Gotto G, Teichman JM. Shock wave lithotripsy correlates with stone density on preoperative computerized tomography. *J Urol.* 2007; 178(3 Pt 1):912-5.

[38] Ouzaid I, Al-Qahtani S, Dominique S, Hupertan V, Fernandez P, Hermieu JF, Delmas V, Ravery V. A 970 Hounsfield units (HU) threshold of kidney stone density on non-contrast computed tomography (NCCT) improves patients' selection for extracorporeal shockwave lithotripsy (ESWL): evidence from a prospective study. *BJU Int.* 2012; 110(11 Pt B): E438-42.

[39] Seitz C, Fajković H, Remzi M, Waldert M, Ozsoy M, Kramer G, Marberger M. Rapid extracorporeal shock wave lithotripsy treatment after a first colic episode correlates with accelerated ureteral stone clearance. *Eur Urol.* 2006;49(6):1099-105; discussion 1105-6.

[40] Lindqvist K, Holmberg G, Peeker R, Grenabo L. Extracorporeal shock-wave lithotripsy or ureteroscopy as primary treatment for ureteric stones: a retrospective study comparing two different treatment strategies. *Scand J Urol Nephrol.* 2006;40(2):113-8.

[41] Osorio L, Lima E, Soares J, Autorino R, Versos R, Lhamas A, Marcelo F. Emergency ureteroscopic management of ureteral stones: why not? *Urology*. 2007;69(1):27-31; discussion 31-3.

[42] Platonov MA, Gillis AM, Kavanagh KM. Pacemakers, implantable cardioverter/defibrillators, and extracorporeal shockwave lithotripsy: evidence-based guidelines for the modern era. *J Endourol* 2008; 22(2):243-7.

[43] Ohmori K, Matsuda T, Horii Y, et al. Effects of shock waves on the mouse fetus. *J Urol* 1994; 151(1):255-8.

[44] Semins MJ, Trock BJ, Matlaga BR. The safety of ureteroscopy during pregnancy: a systematic review and meta-analysis. *J Urol* 2009;181(1);139-43.

[45] Rassweiler J, Rassweiler MC, Frede T, Alken P. Extracorporeal shock wave lithotripsy: An opinion on its future. *Indian J Urol.* 2014; 30(1):73-9.

[46] Rassweiler JJ, Knoll T, Köhrmann KU, McAteer JA, Lingeman JE, Cleveland RO, et al. Shock wave technology and application: An update. *Eur Urol.* 2011;59:784–96.

[47] Pishchalnikov YA, McAteer R, VonderHaar J, Pishchalnikova IV, Williams JC, Evan AP. Detection of significant variation in acoustic output of an electromagnetic lithotripter. *J Urol.* 2006;176:2294–8.

[48] De Sio M, Autorino R, Quarto G, Mordente S, Giugliano F, Di Giacomo F, et al. A new transportable shock-wave lithotripsy machine for managing urinary stones: A single centre experience with a dual-focus lithotriptor. *BJU Int.* 2007;100:1137–41.

[49] Zehnder P, Roth B, Birkhäuser F, Schneider S, Schnutz R, Thalmann GN, et al. A prospective randomized trial comparing the modified HM3 with the Modulith SLX-F2 lithotripter. *Eur Urol.* 2011;59:637–44.

[50] Neisius DA. Clinical experience with the latest generation piezoelectric extracorporeal shockwave lithotripsy system. *Eur Kidney Urol Dis.* 2006:81–3.

[51] Wang R, Faerber GJ, Roberts WW, Morris DS, Wolf JS., Jr Single-center North American experience with Wolf Piezolith 3000 in management of urinary calculi. *Urology.* 2009; 73:958–63.

[52] Ng CF, Mc Loman L, Thompson TJ, Tolley DA. Comparison of 2 generations of piezoelectric lithtriptors using matched pair analysis. *J Urol.* 2004;172:1887–91.

[53] Eisenmenger W, Du XX, Tang C, Zhao S, Wang Y, Rong F, et al. The first clinical results of "wide focus and low-pressure" ESWL. *Ultrasound Med Biol.* 2002; 28:769–74.

[54] Lee JY. Evaluation of the optimal frequency of and pretreatment with shock waves in patients with renal stones. *Korean J Urol.* 2011; 52(11):776–781.

[55] Mazzucchi E. Comparison between two shock wave regimens using frequencies of 60 and 90 impulses per minute for urinary stones. *Clinics (Sao Paulo)* 2010; 65(10):961–965.

[56] Chacko J. Does a slower treatment rate impact the efficacy of extracorporeal shock wave lithotripsy for solitary kidney or ureteral stones? *J Urol.* 2006; 175(4):1370–1373.

[57] Maloney ME. Progressive increase of lithotripter output produces better in vivo stone comminution. *J Endourol.* 2006; 20(9):603–606.

[58] Zhu Y, Duijvesz D, Rovers MM, et al. alpha-Blockers to assist stone clearance after extracorporeal shock wave lithotripsy: a meta-analysis. *BJU Int* 2010; 106(2):256-61.

[59] Zheng S, Liu LR, Yuan HC, et al. Tamsulosin as adjunctive treatment after shockwave lithotripsy in patients with upper urinary tract stones: a systematic review and meta-analysis. *Scand J Urol Nephrol* 2010; 44(6):425-32.

[60] Kanao K. Preoperative nomograms for predicting stone-free rate after extracorporeal shock wave lithotripsy. *J Urol.* 2006; 176:1453–1457.

[61] Nakajima Y, Kanao K. Current topics in the management of urinary tract stones; preoperative nomograms for predicting stone-free rate after ESWL. (Proceedings of 29th annual Jackson Hole Urologic conference, 24 – 30 January 2009, Teton Village, Wyoming, USA).

[62] Vakalopoulos I. Development of a mathematical model to predict extracorporeal shockwave lithotripsy outcome. *J Endourol.* 2009; 23(6):891–897.

[63] Wiesenthal JD. A clinical nomogram to predict the successful shock wave lithotripsy of renal and ureteral calculi. *J Urol.* 2011; 186(2): 556–562.

In: Urolithiasis
Editor: Joseph Fletcher

ISBN: 978-1-63463-500-4

Chapter 4

Hereditary Kidney Stones

Mohammed S. Al-Marhoon*
Urology Division, Department of Surgery,
College of Medicine and Health Sciences Sultan Qaboos University,
Sultanate of Oman

Abstract

Urolithiasis is a common multifactorial problem with multi-effect on the patients' quality of life and an economic burden on the individual and the health system of the country. Various intrinsic and extrinsic factors are associated with the risk for stone formation. Among intrinsic factors are race, sex, and genetics. Finding the cause of urolithiasis or establishing it early in life will reduce the consequence and complications of kidney stone disease and hence reduction of the cost in the treatment by establishing preventative measures in addition to patient education. Genetic factors play an important role in the etiology of urolithiasis as a polygenic (common) or monogenic (rare) forms, however its knowledge and early diagnosis is important to achieve the goals of reducing patient suffering and the economic burdens. This chapter entitled "Hereditary Kidney Stones" is devoted to understanding, early recognition, management and prevention of complications of hereditary urolithasis.

---

* College of Medicine and Health Sciences Sultan Qaboos University, P. O. Box 35, Al-Khoud 123, Sultanate of Oman. Mobile: (+968) 95208801; Fax: (+968) 24143504. E-mail: msalmarhoon@gmail.com/mmarhoon@squ.edu.om.

This topic is important for urologists in practice to have an in depth knowledge about hereditary kidney stones and how to evaluate and manage them in addition to counseling the patients and their families.

Keywords: Urolithiasis, nephrolithiasis, hereditary, genetic, kidney, stones

1. Introduction

Nephrolithiasis is the formation of crystal aggregates in the urinary tract resulting in kidney stones, whereas nephrocalcinosis is the deposition of calcium concretions in the renal parenchyma. Cystinuria is the formation of cystine stones in the kidneys. However, an unrelated condition that should not be confused with cystinuria is cystinosis which is an autosomal recessive disorder characterized by accumulation of the amino acid cystine in lysosomes. In children cystinosis is the major cause of inherited Fanconi syndromc, while in older patients it can mimic idiopathic nephrotic syndrome. [1]

Nephrolithiasis is a common, complex systemic disorder. The prevalence of nephrolithiasis (history of stone disease) varies by age, sex, race, and geography. The prevalence increases with age, and the lifetime risk of stone formation in the USA exceeds 12% in men and 6% in women. [2] The incidence of nephrolithiasis (the first stone event) varies by age, sex, and race. White males have the highest incidence rates. In men, the incidence begins to rise after age 20, peaks between 40 and 60 years at 3/1000/year and then declines. In women, the incidence is higher in their late twenties at 2.5/1000/year and then decreases to 1/1000/year by age 50. [3] The 5-year recurrence rate for stone formation after the initial episode has been suggested at 30-40% of untreated individuals. The risk of recurrence is affected by a variety of factors including stone type and urinary composition. [4] Studies of twins and populations have demonstrated that the common forms of stone disease are heritable. The risk of stone formation is twofold higher in individuals with a family history of stone disease. [5] The increased risk is likely due to both genetic predisposition and environmental exposures like diet. In a cross-sectional Canadian study, individuals of Arabic, West Indian, West Asian, and Latin American descent were more likely to be stone formers than those of European descent. [6] Nephrolithiasis is associated with systemic disorders that promote the formation of calcium containing stones such as: Primary hyperparathyroidism; renal tubular acidosis; and Crohn's disease.

In addition, common conditions such as obesity, gout, and diabetes mellitus, have been linked to nephrolithiasis and formation of calcium oxalate or uric acid stones. [7] Occupations with higher insensible fluid losses, such as a hot environment, increase the risk of stone formation. [8] Dietary intake influences urine composition, nutrients like calcium, animal protein, oxalate, sodium, sucrose, fructose, magnesium, and potassium have been found to play a role in modifying the risk of nephrolithiasis. [7]

Genetic factors paly an important role in the etiology of urolithiasis. There are two forms of genetic involvement in urolithaisis; the common polygenic and the rare monogenic forms. The polygenic idiopathic calcium oxalate urolithaisis is a common disorder affecting 10% of adults, [9] whereas the monogenic disorders affect 2% of adults and 10% of children. [10] Clinical recognition of the monogenic hereditary forms of urolithasis can be challenging, due to their rarity, wide spectrum of disease, expression over the course of a lifetime, from childhood to adulthood, and common things and symptoms among the different disorders including overlap with calcium oxalate urolithaisis. Delays in diagnosis are common with identification of some patients only after the onset of renal failure or when there is disease recurrence in the transplanted kidney after transplantation. [11] The etiology of nephrolithiasis in children has shifted from predominantly infectious to metabolic causes. [12] More than 40% of affected children have identifiable metabolic predispositions for nephrolithiasis. [13] Known hereditary renal diseases that may present with renal stones included autosomal dominant polycystic kidney disease (ADPKD) and Bartter's syndrome (high urine calcium excretion). [14]

Kidney stones are a risk factor for chronic kidney disease (CKD). [15] Kidney stones and CKD are common, affecting 5 and 13% of the adult population, respectively. CKD is a recognized complication of kidney stones as a result of rare hereditary disorders (e.g. Primary hyperoxaluria, Dent disease, 2-8-Hydroxyadeninecrystalluria, Cystinuria). Nephrolithiasis and nephrocalcinosis can lead to progressive loss of glomerular filtration rate (GFR) and end stage renal disease (ESRD) at a young age. In addition, infection stones (struvite) can lead to an obstructive nephropathy with staghorn calculi and are the leading cause of ESRD attributed to nephrolithiasis. [16] Recurrent episodes of obstruction and crystal-specific biological effects on tubular epithelial cells and interstitial renal cells may activate the fibrogenic cascade responsible for the loss of renal parenchyma. In clinical terms, frequent stone relapses, episodes of urinary tract infection and obstruction, number of urological interventions, and size of the gravel are all significantly associated with the risk for renal failure. Percutaneous and extracorporeal urological methods for the treatment of renal stones may also lead to chronic deterioration of renal function, particularly in recurrent stone formers treated with multiple therapeutic sessions. [17] This chapter entitled "Hereditary Kidney Stones" is devoted to understanding, early recognition, management and prevention of complications of hereditary urolithasis.

Table 1.1. Stone components

Stone Components	
Name	Types
Oxalates	Calcium oxalates monohydrate (Whewellite)
	Calcium oxalates dihydrate (Weddellite)
Phosphates	Calcium phosphate (Apatite)
	Calcium hydrogen phosphate (Brushite)
	Magnesium-ammonium phosphate (struvite)
	Octacalcium phosphate
	Whitlockite
	Newberyite
Uric acid and Hydrates	Uric acid
	Uric acid dihydrate
	Uric acid monohydrate
Urates and Purine derivates	Ammonium urate
	Xanthine
	Dihydroxyadenine
Cystine	Cystine

1.1. Types of Kidney Stones

Urinary stones are solid biogenous formations of the urinary system. About 95% of stones are crystalline components and 5% are organic components (matrix or proteins). The known stone components are illustrated in (Table 1.1). [18] In Oman the common stone components are shown in (Table1.2). [19] Stone components can be identified by different methods of stone analysis including: Infrared spectroscopy; X-ray diffraction; Polarization microscopy; and Chemical methods. Infrared spectroscopy is the most accurate method. [14] It is based on the interaction of the infrared light and the molecules in the stone components. The light stimulates atomic vibrations.

The consequence is energy absorption, which results in absorption bands in the infrared spectrum. [18] The advantages of infrared spectroscopy are: Moderate costs; very quick examination using new ATR (attenuated total reflection) technique; examinations of small samples are possible; preparation is very easy using ATR technique; and the ability to detect non-crystalline substances as proteins or fat. However, the disadvantages include: Time-consuming preparation applying the usual tablets technique with potassium bromide; differentiation and qualitative analyses are in some cases difficult, for example in the case of uric acid and purines and calcium phosphates.

Table 1.2. Composition of calculi frequency in Omani patients compared to other Gulf and western countries. [19]

Country / Stone Type	Kuwait (%)	Tunis (%)	Iraq (%)	Oman (%)	USA (%)	France (%)
Calcium Oxalate	72.1	97.4	75.7	73.2	74.8	65.4
Calcium Phosphate	3.1	28.4	56.4	29.1	48.1	14.8
Uric acid	15.4	27.7	19.2	19.5	10.7	8.7
Struvite	5.2	6.0	3.8	1.5	3.9	2.2
Cystine	2.4	1.7	1.3	4.0	2.7	1.3

1.2. Prevalence of Hereditary Kidney Stones

Nephrolithiasis is a common disorder, affecting 10% of individuals in Western countries. [20] The recurrence rate is 50% at 5-10 years; which requires frequent urological treatments, [21] with the consequence of a significant morbidity. A positive family history of nephrolithiasis is reported in 15-20% of stone formers. [5] Nephrolithiasis is unusual in children, with an incidence that has been estimated at 0.15%, [22] much lower than among adults. It is worth noting, however, that as many as 40% of children with nephrolithiasis have a positive family history, suggesting a genetic disorder. Common forms of calcium oxalate nephrolithiasis and idiopathic hypercalciuria are complex polygenic disorders, however, in 50% of cases several genes contribute to their pathogenesis. In addition, [23] there are also a few in frequent or even very rare Mendelian monogenic renal stone conditions (Table 1.3), [24] occurring in 1.9%. [10]

The pointers to inherited disease in renal stone patients include: [24] Early onset; family cases; consanguineous parents; highly-active stone disease (bilateral, multiple stones, frequently recurrent); associated nephrocalcinosis; renal hyperechogenicity; tubular dysfunction and related manifestations (statural growth deficit, polyuria, bone disorders); renal failure; extrarenal manifestations (sensorineural hearing defects, ocular abnormalities, neurological disorders); particular stone composition and crystalluria (monohydrate calcium oxalate whewellite; Cystine; Dihydroxyadenine; Xanthine). Consanguinity (which may be quite widespread in some cultures) is also an issue because having a common ancestor raises the risk of developing recessive monogenic diseases. If parents are first cousins, the risk is twice as high as in the offspring of unrelated parents. [25]

1.3. Future Perspectives

Further understanding of the molecular biology and genetics of urinary stones will be the road to specific diagnostic methods based on identifying the concerned genes as well as having specific treatments based on the underlying processes and pathways.

2. Cystinuria

2.1. Introduction

Cystinuria is a rare but an important genetic cause for kidney stones. Patients affected by cystinuria suffer from recurrent stone formation, leading to repeated surgical interventions, renal impairment, and, consequently, significant impairment of life quality. Cystinuria is the result of a defect in proximal tubular reabsorption of filtered cystine, a homodimer of the aminoacid cysteine. [26] The stones are composed of the poorly soluble amino acid cystine. Concomitant loss of ornithine, arginine, and lysine also occur but is not clinically significant. [26]

Table 1.3. Monogenic renal stone diseases. AD: Autosomal dominant; AR: Autosomal recessive; NC: Nephrocalcinosis; ESRD: End stage renal disease. Modified from [24]

	Abnormal protein	Inheritance	Stone composition	Risk of NC	Risk of ESRD
Cystinuria	rBAT or b0,+ AT	AR	Cystine	No	Yes
Dent' s disease	Cl− /H+ exchanger (ClC-5) or phosphatidyl inositolbiphosphate 5-phosphatase	X-linked recessive	Calcium phosphate	Yes	Yes
Familial hypomagnesaemia with hypercalciuria and nephrocalcinosis	Claudin 16	AR	Calcium salts	Yes	Yes
Autosomal-dominant hypocalcaemic hypercalciuria	Calcium-sensing receptor (CaSR)	AD	Calcium salts	Yes	Yes
Distal renal tubular Acidosis (dRTA)	AE1 (anion exchange protein 1), or ATP6V1B1 or ATP6VOA4 subunits of the H+ ATPase ion pump	AD	Calcium phosphate (Apatite)	Yes	Yes
Primary hyperoxaluria Type 1 (PH1)	Liver-specific peroxisomal alanine/glyoxylate aminotransferase	AR	calcium oxalate monohydrated (whewellite)	Yes	Yes
Primary hyperoxaluria Type 2 (PH2)	Glyoxylatereductase/ hydroxypyruvatereductase	AR	calcium oxalate monohydrated (whewellite)	Yes	Yes

Table 3.1. (Continued)

	Abnormal protein	Inheritance	Stone composition	Risk of NC	Risk of ESRD
Primary hyperoxaluria Type 3 (PH3)	Mitochondrial 4-hydroxy-2-oxoglutarate aldolase	AR	Pure monohydrated calcium oxalate (whewellite)	Yes	Yes
Hypoxanthineguanine phosphoribosyltransferase (HGPRT) deficiency (Lesch-Nyhan syndrome)	HGPRT	X-linked Recessive	Uric acid	No	Yes
Phosphoribosyl Pyrophosphatesynthase (PRPPS) hyperactivity	PRPPS	X-linked	Uric acid	No	Yes
Xanthine oxidase Deficiency (xanthinuria)	Xanthine oxidase or molybdenum cofactor sulfurase	AR	Xanthine	No	Yes
Dihydroxyadeninuria (DHA)	Adenine phosphoribosyltransferase (APRT)	AR	Dihydroxyadenine	Yes	Yes

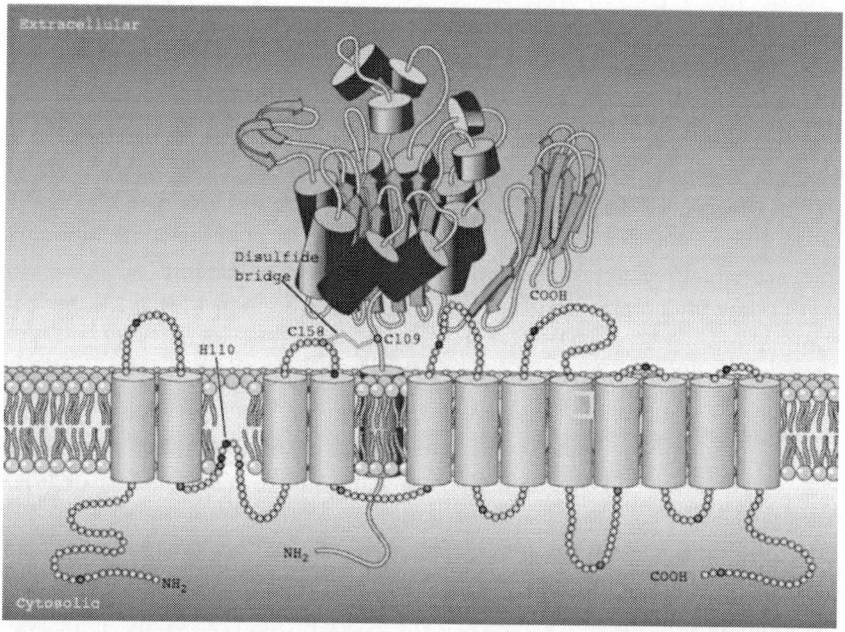

Figure 2.1. The cystine heterodimeric aminoacid transporter. The heavy subunit (pink) and the light subunit (blue) are linked by a disulfide bridge (yellow). Diagram from Reference [7].

2.2. Prevalence

Cystinuria accounts for 1-2% of all renal stones, and 10-25% of childhood stone disease. [27, 28] The worldwide prevalence of cystinuria is estimated at 1:7,000, ranging from 1:2500 among a population of Libyan Jews [26] to 1:100,000 persons in Sweden. In the United States, cystinuria occurs in approximately1:15,000 adults. [29] In Oman cystinuria has been found to account for 4% of adult stones. [30]

2.3. Genetics

The responsible genes causing cystinuria were first described in 1994. [31] Cystinuria is an autosomal-recessive genetic disorder. Two genes *SLC3A1* and *SLC7A9* are proven to be involved, [32] whose protein products are required for the tubular transport of cystine reabsorption, each gene is coding for a subunit of a heterodimeric amino acid transporter situated at the brush border of the proximal tubule and in the gastrointestinal tract. The gene *SLC3A1* situated on chromosome 2 (2p16.3) codes for the heavy rBAT subunit (related to b0,+AT amino acid transporter). Whereas, the gene *SLC7A9* situated on chromosome 19 (19q12–13) codes for the light b0,+AT subunit (amino acid transporter of positively charged or neutral amino acids). Cystine transporter is composed of two subunits: The hydrophobic light subunit (50 kDa) with 12 transmembrane domains and the heavy subunit (80 kDa) with a large extracellular part and one transmembrane domain that are linked by a disulfide bridge (Figure 2.1). Mutation of both alleles of *SLC3A1* or*SLC7A9* will lead to failure of reabsorption of filtered cystine at the glomerulus and excretion of abnormal amounts of the insoluble cystine. Heterozygous for *SLC3A1* mutations usually do not have cystine in the urine, while heterozygotes for *SLC7A9* mutations will have abnormal amounts of urinary cysteine that are very rarely sufficient to cause stones.

Cystinuria is classified into three types: Type A cystinuria (45.2%) is the result of mutations in both *SLC3A1* alleles and type B (53.2%) is the result of mutations in both *SLC7A9* alleles. Type AB patients (1.6%) are homozygous for mutations in either *SLC3A1* or *SLC7A9*. [33]

2.4. Presentation

Most patients with cystinuria present in childhood with recurrent urinary tract stones. Males are affected more than females. [34] The average age of detection of a first renal stone is 12 years [34] with 50% forming a first stone in the first decade of life and another 25% in teenage years. In hypotonia-cystinuria syndrome (mutations of both *SLC3A1* and the contiguous gene *PREPL*, prolylendopeptidase-like protein) children have cystinuria, severe hypotonia at birth, delayed growth and hyperphagia and excessive weight gain later in childhood. [35] A significant proportion of adults with cystinuria develop chronic kidney disease and the renal pathologic findings correlate with the reduction in GFR. [36]

2.5. Complications

Recurrent stone formation, obstructive uropathy and repeated surgical interventions may lead to kidney damage and chronic kidney disease.

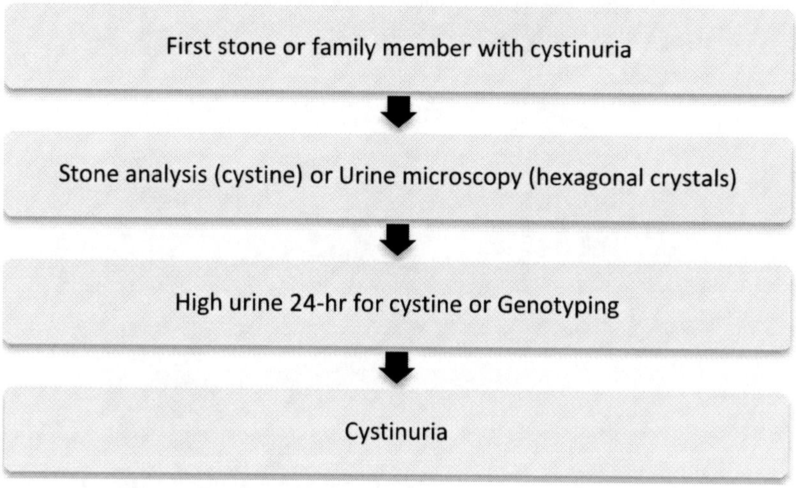

Figure 2.2. Cystinuria diagnostic algorithm.

2.6. Diagnosis

A simplified diagnostic algorithm for cystinuria is presented in Figure 2.2. Cystine stones have an amber color and a waxy appearance (Figure 2.3). Due to the rapid growth they often present as staghorn stones at first diagnosis. Demonstration of hexagonal crystals on urinalysis is pathognomonic of cystinuria (Figure 2.4).

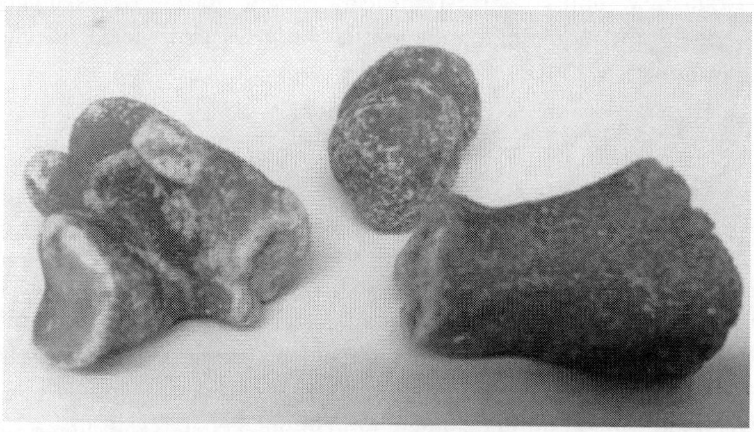

Figure 2.3. Cystine stones. Picture from Dr. Al-Marhoon stone analysis laboratory.

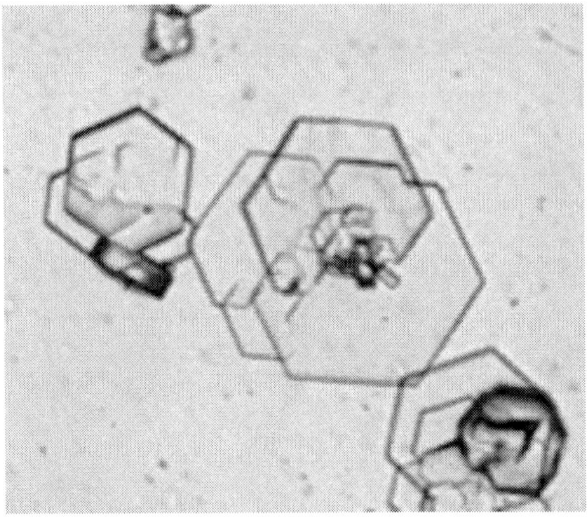

Figure 2.4. Urinary cystine crystal. The typical 6-sided crystal is diagnostic of cystinuria. Picture form Reference. [7].

Cystinuria is diagnosed by demonstration of a cystine stone in a patient (stone analysis), and increased urinary excretion of cystine, or identification of mutations on both alleles of one of the two genes involved. [37] A patient can be considered having cystinuria in the absence of a urinary stone if urine cystine excretion exceeds 1300 micromol/g creatinine (150 mmol/mmol creatinine). On radiography, cystine stones present as poorly radiopaque, while in computed tomography (CT) scans, cystine stones have poor attenuation of 860 Hounsfield units. [38] At present, genetic testing for patients with cystinuria is not required for diagnostic purposes and yields no clinically useful information. [39].

2.7. Treatment

Treatment of cystinuria focuses on reducing the supersaturation of urinary cystine to limit the potential of crystallization. The variables that can be addressed include cystine concentration, cysteine amount and urine pH. Oral fluid intake of 3 l/day, as tolerated, should be prescribed to decrease urine cystine concentration to less than 250 mg/l (about 1 mmol/l). Dietary manipulations like limiting animal protein intake and salt ingestion may reduce the amount of excreted cysteine. [40] Cystine supersaturation is significantly reduced at higher urine pH. The goal of therapy is to alkalinize the urine to pH of 7.5 with potassium citrate. Sodium citrate should be avoided because of the effect of increased urine sodium on urine cystine excretion. When fluid intake and alkalinization fail to halt stone formation, the thiol drugs D-penicillamine and tiopronin are both efficacious at breaking the disulfide bridge of cystine and forming soluble drug-cysteine complexes. [41] Significant side effects, including rash, allergy, hematologic and liver function abnormalities and rarely nephrotic syndrome due to membranous nephropathy are associated with using the thiol drugs. It has been shown that adapting the prophylactic regimens can reduce stone recurrence. [42]

Most cystinuria patients require multiple urological interventions during their lifetime. [43] Cystine stones are often less amenable to being broken by shockwave lithotripsy, but can be turned to dust by ureteroscopy and the holmium laser. [44] However, shockwave lithotripsy has been shown to be effective for cystine stones in children more than adults. [45] Open surgery for kidney stones may be considered for staghorn stones.

2.8. Prognosis

Incidence of stone formation in the affected population varies between 0.2 and 0.8 stone events/year. [41] A 5-year recurrence rate of 73%, independent of the amount of urinary cystine, type of intervention, or presence of residual calculi, has been described. [41] The repeated stone formation leading to repeated interventions may lead to renal impairment in up to 70%. End stage renal disease may occur in up to 5%, unilateral nephrectomy in up to 15%. [17]

2.9. Conclusion

Cystine stones are important hereditary stones that are amenable to medical and surgical management. Early diagnosis is crucial for the following reasons: Reduced kidney damage by repeated urological interventions; improve the patient quality of life; and screen the patient family members for the disease. The main goal of conservative management is the improvement of the solubility of urinary cystine that can be achieved by dietary measures, leading to a decrease of urinary cystine concentration, and drugs leading to reduction of cystine to the more soluble cysteine. Continuous education of the patient and his family about the disease and its consequences and the methods for its prevention are essential for an effective management.

3. Hypercalciuria

3.1. Introduction

Hypercalciuria is defined as the excretion of urinary calcium exceeding 200 mg/24-h. There are three forms of hypercalciuria: Absorptive hypercalciuria (intestinal hyperabsorption of calcium); Renal hypercalciuria (renal leak of calcium), and Resorptive hypercalciuria (increased bone resorption associated with primary hyperparathyroidism). [7] Hypercalciuria can be caused by defects in various genes (polygenic) or a single gene (monogenic), which can be passed on to family members and can cause stones. The polygenic hypercalciuria (idiopathic) is the underlying cause of kidney stones in 60% of the common idiopathic calcium oxalate urolithaisis. [11] However, the monogenic hypercalciuria is the underlying cause of several rare conditions promoting the formation of calcium stones. They include: Hereditary distal renal tubular acidosis; Dent disease; Autosomal dominant hypocalcemic hypercalciuria; and familial hypomagnesemia with hypercalciuria and nephrocalcinosis (FHHNC).

3.2. Prevalence

The polygenic idiopathic calcium oxalate urolithaisis is a common disorder affecting 10% of adults, [9] whereas the monogenic disorders affect 2% of adults and 10% of children. [10] Dent disease is a rare renal tubular disorder, with about 250 affected families having been reported around the world. [7]

3.3. Genetics

Idiopathic calcium oxalate urolithaisis, arises from a combination of environmental factors including the dietary intake of salts, protein, calcium, and fluid, in addition to climate and socioeconomic status as well as genetic factors where a member of the claudin gen family (CLDN14) has been identified as a risk locus. [46] The complexity of the underlying physiological defects, which may affect kidney, intestine, and bone, has complicated the search for gene defects linked with this disorder. However, in spite of this complexity, a number of gene defects have been discovered for the absorptive hypercalciuria including: Polymorphisms of the vitamin D receptor (VDR) gene defects; [47] base substitutions in the adenylatecyclase gene (AHRAC); [48] and polymorphism in the calcitonin receptor gene. [49] Mutation of the calcium-sensing receptor (CASR) has been associated with several familial syndromes related to hypercalciuria with stone formation. The CASR is a plasma membrane G protein-coupled receptor in the parathyroid gland responsible for detecting changes in Ca^{2+} concentration and modifying parathyroid hormone (PTH) secretion and renal cation handling. The gene encoding the CASR has been mapped to chromosome 3q13.3-q2. [50]

Dent disease was described in 1990 as a group of X-linked renal disorders characterized by low-molecular-weight proteinuria, and variable presence of hypercalciuria, nephrocalcinosis and nephrolithiasis. It is caused by mutations in the *CLCN5* gene, located on the X chromosome (Xp11.22). This gene encodes a 746-amino-acid voltage-gated chloride channels (CLC-5). [51] In the human kidney, CLC-5 is primarily expressed in proximal tubular cells, alpha- and beta-intercalated cells of the cortical collecting duct, and in the thick ascending limb of Henle's loop. [52] In proximal tubular cells it is involved in the endocytic reabsorption of low-molecular-weight proteins that have passed the glomerular filter. Specifically, CLC-5 has been proposed to function by providing a shunt conductance in early endosomes, thus permitting their efficient intraluminal acidification by a V-type H+-ATPase. [52] Defective recycling of low-molecular-weight proteins explains the low-molecular-weight proteinuria in affected patients. However, hypercalciuria and stone formation have been suggested to arise from secondary effects of defective endocytic transport. Tow postulates have been suggested: Decreased endocytosis of PTH results in increased stimulation of PTH receptors, with consequent stimulation of hydroxylation of 25-hydroxy vitamin D3 to its active form; [53] and impaired internalization of the calcium channel (EcaC). [54] However, 15% of patients with Dent disease, which is now termed Dent 2 disease, are caused by *OCRL1* mutations. [55] *OCRL1* encodes a phosphatidylinositol 4,5-biphosphate 5-phosphatase localized at the Golgi apparatus.

Familial hypomagnesemia with hypercalciuria and nephrocalcinosis (FHHNC) is a rare autosomal recessive disorder characterized by renal magnesium wasting, hypercalciuria, nephrocalcinosis and kidney failure. The disease was first described in 1972 [56] and hypomagnesemia is a characteristic feature of the disease, [57] which is due to impairment in the reabsorption of magnesium and calcium in the thick ascending limb of the loop of Henle. [58] The molecular defect is caused by mutations in two genes, *CLDN16* located on the chromosome 3q27 and *CLDN19* on chromosome 1p34.2. [59] The proteins encoded by these two genes, claudin-16 and claudin-19, are integral membrane proteins that are involved in paracellular reabsorption of calcium and magnesium. [60] The reported median age at onset of symptoms ranges from 3.5 to 7 years. [57]

Distal renal tubular acidosis (dRTA) type 1 has impairment in hydrogen-ion secretion in the distal nephron, leading to a metabolic acidosis and often hypokalemia. Stones formed are composed of calcium phosphate and result from a number of urinary abnormalities, including increased urinary calcium and phosphate excretion, high urinary pH, and decreased excretion of citrate. [61] Both autosomal dominant and recessive inheritance patterns occur with more severe phenotype and earlier onset associated with the recessive form of the disorder. Mutations of the genes *AE1*; *ATP6B1*; and *ATP6NB1* have been reported. [62]

3.4. Presentation

Stones formed by Dent disease patients are composed of calcium oxalate or calcium phosphate. Clinically the presentation of disease is variable, which lead to the description of three separate syndromes of X-linked nephrolithiasis, Dent's disease, hypophosphatemic rickets type III, and idiopathic low-molecular-weight (LMW) proteinuria. [63] Dent disease usually presents with LMW proteinuria and hypercalciuria in childhood or early adult life with males much more severely affected than females. [63] Other presenting features in children and adolescents often include hematuria, nephrocalcinosis and hypercalciuria, with or without kidney stones. It must be stressed that LMW proteinuria is the pathognomonic feature of Dent disease, and can occur in isolation. [64]

The most common presenting features of FHHNC are recurrent urinary tract infection, polyuria and polydipsia, hematuria and pyuria. [57] Additional manifestations at onset include kidney stones, failure to thrive, seizures, abdominal pain and muscular tetany due to symptomatic hypocalcemia or hypomagnesemia. All affected patients have hypomagnesemia, hypercalciuria and nephrocalcinosis at the time of diagnosis. Other notable biochemical abnormalities observed during the course of the disease are hypocalcemia, incomplete distal renal tubular acidosis, hypocitraturia, increased parathyroid hormone levels independent of GFR and hyperuricemia. Approximately 30% of patients experience episodes of kidney stones. [65] Occasionaly proteinuria has been reported in patients with FHHNC. Ocular findings in patients with *CLDN19* mutations include myopia, pigmentary retinitis, macular coloboma, strabismus, astigmatism and nystagmus. [66] The diagnosis of FHHNC should be considered in all children with nephrocalcinosis, history of kidney stones, and/or reduced kidney function.

Distal renal tubular acidosis (dRTA) type 1 is associated with nephrocalcinosis or nephrolithiasis. [67] In familial dRTA, affected children usually present with failure to thrive and growth retardation. Both autosomal dominant and recessive inheritance patterns occur with more severe phenotype and earlier onset associated with the recessive form of the disorder. The recessive form of dRTA is frequently accompanied by sensorineural hearing loss.

3.5. Complications

Dent disease is associated with the development of CKD. Most patients are recognized due to the presence of nephrocalcinosis or unexplained CKD, hypophosphatemia and bone disease. More recently, patients have been recognized with nephrotic-range proteinuria and glomerular changes of focal segmental glomerulosclerosis (FSGS) on renal biopsy. [64] In FHHNC chronic kidney disease is frequently present in childhood with one-third of patients reaching ESRD during adolescence. [66]

3.6. Diagnosis

Diagnostic features of Dent disease include LMW proteinuria (β2 microglobulin, α1 microglobulin, or retinol binding protein), hypercalciuria, nephrolithiasis or nephrocalcinosis and renal insufficiency. Dent disease cases have been reported with LMW proteinuria alone. However, one or more of the following additional features is sufficient to make a clinical diagnosis of Dent disease when LMW proteinuria is present: Stones or nephrocalcinosis, hypercalciuria, hypophosphatemia with or without rickets, or a family history of Dent disease. Genetic screening of the two implicated genes (*CLCN5* and *OCRL1*) can be confirmatory. Findings on renal biopsy consistent with Dent disease include nephrocalcinosis, interstitial fibrosis, and focal segmental glomerulosclerosis. [64] The outline of diagnostic algorithm for dent disease is presented in Figure 3.1.

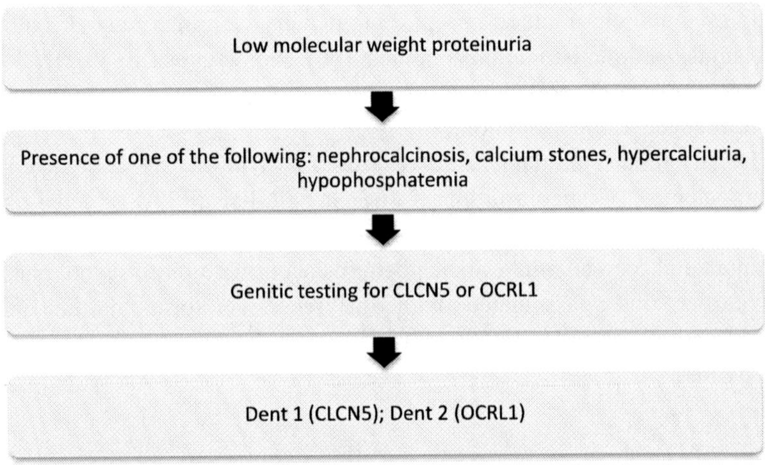

Figure 3.1. Dent disease diagnostic algorithm.

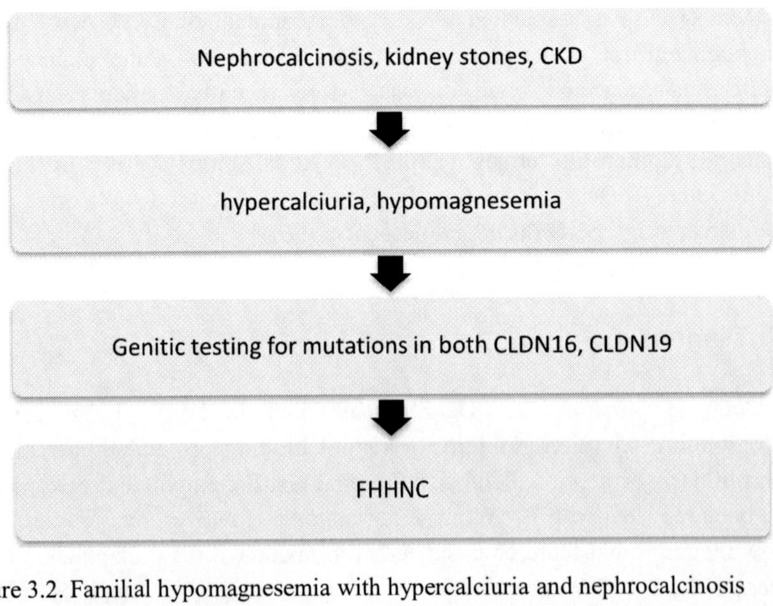

Figure 3.2. Familial hypomagnesemia with hypercalciuria and nephrocalcinosis (FHHNC) diagnostic algorithm.

The diagnosis of FHHNC is based on the triad of hypomagnesemia, hypercalciuria and nephrocalcinosis with or without hypocalcemia, incomplete distal renal tubular acidosis and hypocitraturia. [68] Levels of serum magnesium and urinary calcium should be measured in all patients with nephrocalcinosis and/or CKD. High fractional urinary excretion of magnesium is found while serum magnesium is inappropriately low. [69] Urinary calcium-to-creatinine ratio can be used to estimate the urinary calcium excretion. Renal histologic findings are not specific and include calcium deposits, glomerulosclerosis, tubular atrophy and interstitial fibrosis, consistent with a chronic tubulointerstitial nephropathy. In the differential diagnosis, the presence of CKD distinguishes FHHNC from other magnesium wasting disorders. Excluding hypokalemic metabolic alkalosis is important in the diagnostic process to avoid confusion with Bartter syndrome. The diagnosis of FHHNC can be confirmed by demonstrating mutations in both copies of *CLDN16* or *CLDN19*. The outline of diagnostic algorithm for FHHNC is presented in Figure 3.2. An outline for the diagnostic algorithm of distal renal tubular acidosis (dRTA) is presented in Figure 3.3.

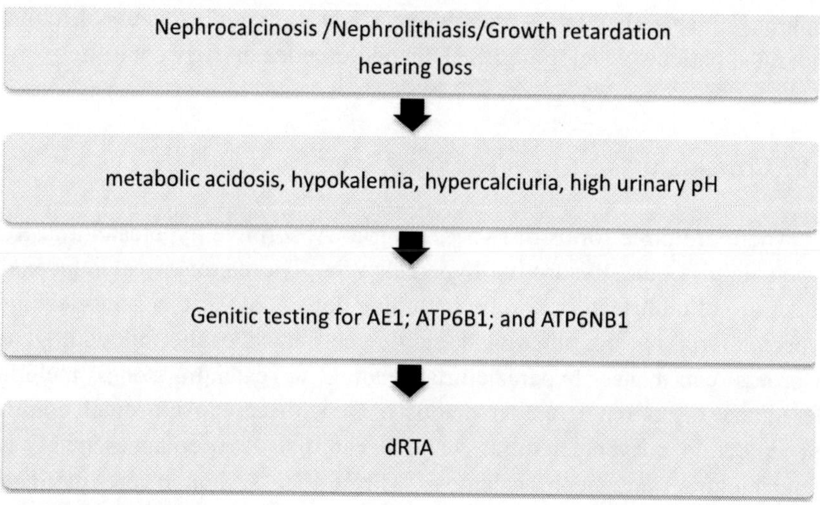

Figure 3.3. Distal renal tubular acidosis (dRTA) diagnostic algorithm.

3.7. Treatment

In Dent disease, Stones, when present, are composed of calcium oxalate and/or calcium phosphate. There is no treatment that targets the specific defect causing Dent disease. The primary goal of treatment, therefore, is delaying the progression of CKD. Available interventions are primarily aimed at decreasing hypercalciuria and preventing kidney stones and nephrocalcinosis. Thiazide diuretics used to treat kidney stone disease as they decrease urinary calcium excretion, and Angiotensin-converting enzyme (ACE) inhibitors and angiotensin receptor blockers (ARB) used in children with proteinuria to prevent or delay further loss of kidney function, and a high citrate diet to slow progression of CKD have been tried. [70]

Medical management of FHHNC has included administration of magnesium supplements in high doses and thiazide diuretics to reduce urinary calcium excretion and the progression of nephrocalcinosis. [69] However, no effective therapeutic interventions for FHHNC are available.

3.8. Prognosis

In Dent disease 30–80% of affected males progress to CKD in their 3rd and 5th decades of life. In familial hypomagnesemia with hypercalciuria and nephrocalcinosis (FHHNC) progressive CKD commonly occurs in children with most patients developing ESRD in adolescence or early adult life.

3.9. Conclusion

There are three forms of hypercalciuria: Absorptive hypercalciuria; Renal hypercalciuria, and Resorptive hypercalciuria. The common calcium oxalate stones are of multifactorial origin including defects of various genes leading to hypercalciuria. On the other hand, single gen defects of the following genetic disorders can cause hypercalciuria leading to calcium stones including: Hereditary distal renal tubular acidosis; Dent disease; Autosomal dominant hypocalcemic hypercalciuria; and Familial hypomagnesemia with hypercalciuria and nephrocalcinosis (FHHNC). Although the monogenic disorders are rare but they are characterized by more severe progressive renal impairment than the common polygenic form.

4. Primary Hyperoxaluria

4.1. Introduction

The primary hyperoxaluria (PH) are inherited disorders of metabolism in which hepatic enzyme deficiencies result in overproduction of oxalate. The excess oxalate cannot be degraded in humans and is excreted largely by the kidneys, resulting in high urinary concentrations. Calcium oxalate crystals form in renal tubules acting as a nidus for crystal aggregation and growth, thus initiating stone formation. Crystals attach to renal tubular epithelial cells causing degenerative change, necrosis and inflammatory reaction leading to renal injury and scarring. [71] Health consequences include frequent formation of calcium oxalate kidney stones as well as renal injury that leads to kidney failure in a significant proportion of affected patients. [72]

4.2. Prevalence

Primary hyperoxaluria is worldwide in its distribution. In central Europe the incidence of 1:120,000 live births and prevalence of 1-3 per million population has been reported. [73] The prevalence of PH appears to be higher in certain regions including the Canary Islands, Tunisia, and parts of the Middle East. [73]

4.3. Genetics

Three types of primary hyperoxaluria (PH) have been described, each involving a different enzyme of the oxalate metabolic pathways in the liver. Type 1 PH (80% of patients) an autosomal recessive disease is due to mutations in the gene AGXT found in chromosome 2q36-37. When the activity of alanine-glyoxylate aminotransferase (AGT) is reduced or absent, glyoxylate accumulates and is shunted to oxalate and glycolate. For effective disposition of glyoxylate, AGT must be present in the peroxisome of the hepatocyte. Mistargeting of AGT to mitochondria, as results from certain mutations in AGXT, also results in hyperoxaluria even though enzyme activity is measurable. [74] Type 2 PH (10% of patients) an autosomal dominant diseases is caused by mutations in the enzyme glyoxylatereductase/hydroxy pyruvate reductase (GRHPR). [75] Type 3 PH (10% of patients) is caused by mutations of the enzyme 4-hydroxy-2-oxaloglutarate aldolase (HOGA1) found in hepatic mitochondria. [76]

4.4. Presentation

Some children initially present with failure to thrive, nausea, pallor or fatigue of ESRD with no history of stones. Such patients may have diffuse calcification of kidney tissue (nephrocalcinosis) visible by ultrasound or other imaging studies without discrete stones. Extensive calcium oxalate crystal deposition is observed on renal biopsy. This mode of presentation is seen especially in infants. Irreversible kidney failure can be evident as early as 4 months of age. Recurring stones throughout childhood, adolescence, and adulthood are characteristic. Growth and development are normal unless compromised by CKD or other unrelated medical problems. Over time, however, progressive renal damage leads to reduced kidney function. Effects on kidney function vary by type, with PH1 the most severe. Patients with PH2 and PH3 appear to have better kidney outcomes. In adults, most patients present with signs or symptoms related to kidney stones.

4.5. Complications

Nephrocalcinosis or nephrolithiasis leading to chronic kidney disease (CKD) and end stage renal disease (ESRD) are the feared complications.

4.6. Diagnosis

The diagnosis of PH should be suspected in any child or adolescent who presents with radiopaque stones consistent with calcium oxalate, especially if stones are bilateral or present before a child is of school age. Stone analysis and 24 h urine collection are essential. The stones are typically calcium oxalate monohydrate and occasionally composed of mixed calcium oxalate monohydrate with calcium oxalate dehydrate. The diagnosis of PH can be confirmed by DNA testing. However, delays in diagnosis have unwanted consequences including: Delaying effective therapy, impaired renal function, and systemic oxalosis that can cause risk of allograft loss after kidney transplantation. An outline of the diagnostic algorithm for PH is presented in Figure 4.1.

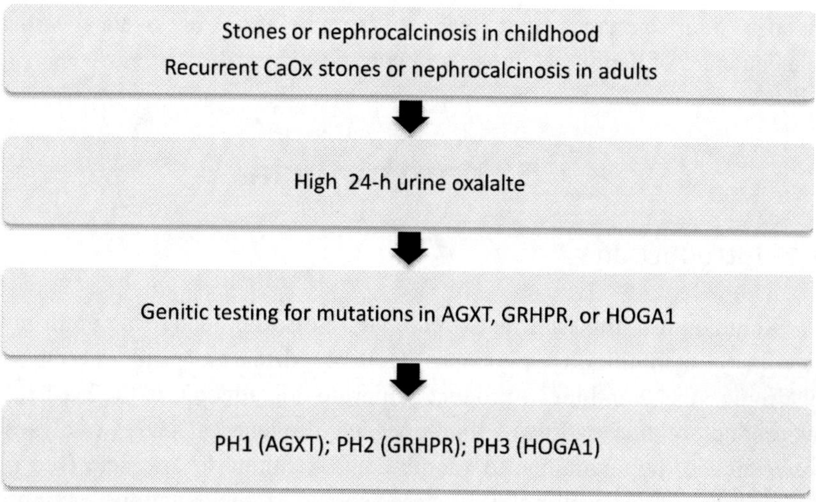

Figure 4.1. Diagnostic algorithm for Primary hyperoxaluria (PH). CaOx: Calcium oxalate; 24-h: 24-hour urine collection of oxalate.

4.7. Treatment

Treatment of primary hyperoxaluria is aimed at decreasing oxalate production and increasing urinary solubility of calcium oxalate. The following therapies have been advocated: Increasing fluid intake, pyridoxine, [77] orthophosphate, [78] magnesium oxide, potassium citrate, [79] and sodium citrate. However, in patients with progressive renal damage leading to failure, combined renal and liver transplantation are recommended. The role of enteric elimination of oxalate by treatment with oral Oxalobacter formigenes might reduce oxalate absorption and promote its secretion into the intestinal lumen. [78] However, a recent double blind, placebo controlled clinical trial conducted failed to show benefit. [80]

4.8. Prognosis

Complications such as chronic kidney disease and failure of transplanted kidney can occur if left untreated.

4.9. Conclusion

Primary hyperoxaluria is an inherited disease due to deficiencies in specific liver enzymes that lead to accumulation of oxalate with the consequences of nephrocalcinosis and chronic kidney disease.

5. Xanthinuria

5.1. Introduction

Xanthine urolithiasis is an extremely rare disorder, occurring in those with hereditary xanthinuria, myeloproliferative diseases, and Lesch-Nyhan syndrome. [81] Xanthine, a product of purine degradation, is the least soluble by product of this pathway. Xanthine dehydrogenase (XDH) catalyzes the conversion of hypoxanthine to xanthine and xanthine to uric acid (see figure 6.1, section 6). Allopurinol is a stereoisomer of hypoxanthine, acting as a competitive inhibitor of XDH. This medication is used as a common treatment for gout and other hyperuricemic states. Allopurinol reduces uric acid production and generates xanthine and hypoxanthine, which are either excreted in the urine or recycled by the hypoxanthine-guanine-phosphoribosyltransferase pathway. Stone formation may occur in those in whom urine is supersaturated with xanthine. Xanthine calculi typically develop in acidic urine.

5.2. Prevalence

The incidence of hereditary xanthinuria is estimated to be between 1:6000 and 1:69,000. [82]

5.3. Genetics

There are two types of hereditary xanthinuria. Both are autosomal recessive disorders with similar clinical manifestations. Type I is due to a deficiency in the activity of xanthine dehydrogenase (XDH) and its gene localized to chromosome 2p22-23. [83] Type II is due to deficiencies in XDH and aldehyde dehydrogenase.

5.4. Presentation

Xanthine stones typically occur in the upper urinary tract, but bladder stones can occur. Approximately 40% of those afflicted develop nephrolithiasis, and the disease typically manifests in childhood. [84] Hypouricemia, reduced urinary uric acid, and increased urinary xanthine excretion are seen. Patients receiving allopurinol therapy to reduce hyperuricemia, those undergoing systemic chemotherapy for myeloproliferative disorders, and those afflicted with Lesch-Nyhan syndrome may develop xanthine stones. Patients with Lesch-Nyhan syndrome are retarded and exhibit self-mutilation and choreoathetosis. This condition is an X-linked disorder caused by a deficiency in hypoxanthine-guanine-phosphoribosyltransferase. Resultant urate overproduction can lead to gouty arthritis and uric acid nephrolithiasis. Fatal uric acid nephropathy may develop. Therefore, allopurinol therapy is routinely administered, because it promotes xanthine and hypoxanthine accumulation, accentuated by the defect in hypoxanthine-guanine-phosphoribosyltransferase. The solubility of hypoxanthine in urine is high, but it is low for xanthine. Thus, these patients have a risk of developing xanthine stones. [81] Cases of patients with Lesch-Nyhan syndrome developing renal failure because of uric acid nephropathy or stone obstruction have been reported. [85]

5.5. Complications

Nephrolithiasis and nephropathy are the consequences.

5.6. Diagnosis

Xanthine stones are usually radiolucent on standard imaging and have attenuation values similar to uric acid on computed tomography. These radiographic characteristics may lead to an initial diagnosis of uric acid nephrolithiasis.

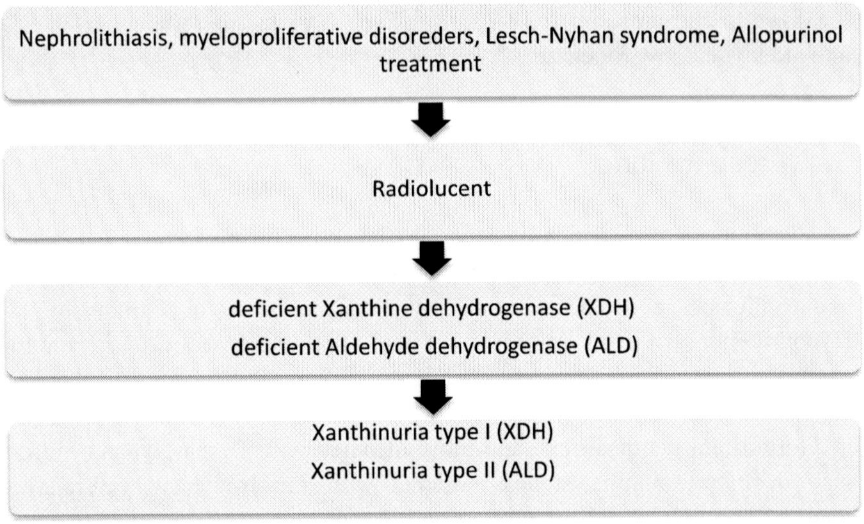

Figure 5.1. Xanthinuria diagnostic algorithm.

5.7. Treatment

The mainstays for treating patients with xanthine nephrolithiasis are aggressive hydration, urinary pH manipulation, and alterations in the allopurinol dose. [86] Xanthinuria is primarily a hepatic disease because XDH is found predominately in the liver and as such, specific attention should be given to the hepatic defect when treating the presenting renal disease.

5.8. Prognosis

Nephrolitiahsis with its complications are the consequences.

5.9. Conclusion

Xanthine urolithiasis is an extremely rare disorder due to deficiency of specific liver enzymes. The radiolucent xanthine stones can be confused with uric acid stones.

6. Dihydroxyadeninuria

6.1. Introduction

Adenine phosphoribosyltransferase (APRT) deficiency is a rare autosomal recessive inborn error of adenine metabolism resulting in the generation of large amounts of the poorly soluble Dihydroxyadenin (DHA), which leads to stone formation in the urinary tract and crystalline nephropathy. [87]

6.2. Prevalence

APRT deficiency was first described in 1968. [88] Subsequently, it has since been described in all ethnic groups, although the majority of reported cases have come from Japan, France, and Iceland. [87]

6.3. Genetics

In adenine phosphoribosyltransferase (APRT) deficiency, adenine cannot be converted to adenosine monophosphate and is instead converted by xanthine dehydrogenase to 2,8-dihydroxyadenine (Figure 6.1). [39] The human APRT gene, located on chromosome 16q24, is 2,466 base pairs long and contains five exons encoding a180 amino acid protein. [89] More than 40 functionally significant human APRT mutations that completely abolish the function of the enzyme in vivo have been reported. Most of these mutations are single base changes and small deletions. The estimated heterozygote frequency in different populations ranges from 0.4 to 1.2%, [90] suggesting that the prevalence of a homozygous state is at least 1:50,000-100,000.

6.4. Presentation

Radiolucent kidney stones are by far the most common clinical manifestation of APRT deficiency in the pediatric population. [87] An initial presentation of acute kidney injury due to bilateral DHA calculi causing urinary tract obstruction has also been documented in children. [91] Other common clinical features include recurrent urinary tract infections, hematuria, and reddish-brown diaper stain. [92] However, some children remain asymptomatic throughout childhood and, not uncommonly, the disease is diagnosed by the detection of DHA crystals on routine urine microscopy or through screening of siblings of index cases. [93]

6.5. Complications

Although CKD with reduced glomerular filtration rate (GFR) has been reported in a number of children with APRT deficiency, ESRD secondary to crystalline nephropathy is a much more common presenting feature of APRT deficiency in adults, [87] which in a number of cases has not been recognized until after kidney transplantation has been performed. [94] There is suggestive evidence that APRT deficiency may be a seriously under recognized cause of kidney stones and CKD that progresses to ESRD in a significant proportion of untreated patients. [94]

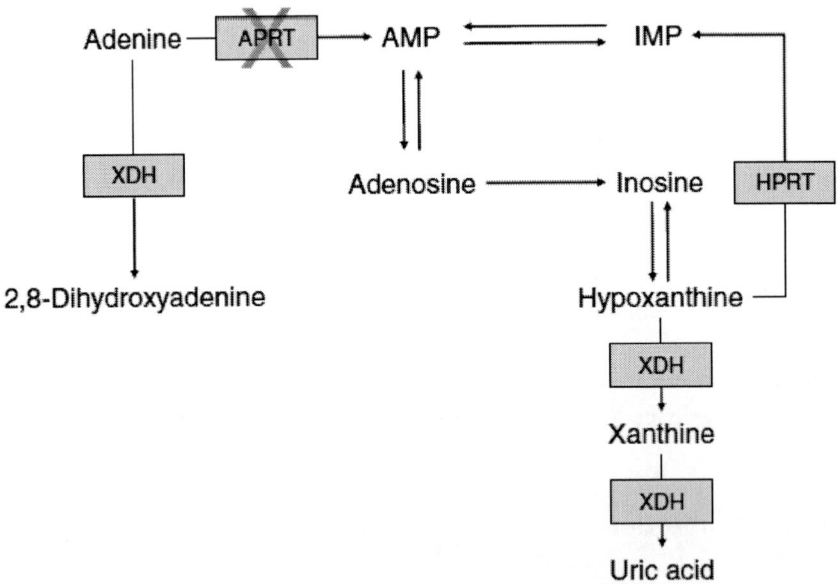

Figure 6.1. Schematic diagram of adenine metabolism. Diagram from reference. [39] APRT, adenine phosphoribosyltransferase; AMP, adenosine monophosphate; HPRT, hypoxanthine-guanine phosphoribosyltransferase; IMP, inosine monophosphate; XDH, xanthine dehydrogenase.

6.6. Diagnosis

The diagnosis of APRT deficiency should be considered in all children presenting with renal colic, radiolucent kidney stones or acute kidney injury and in infants with a history of reddish-brown diaper stain. [87] It is particularly important to consider APRT deficiency in children with radiolucent stones because uric acid stones are uncommon in this age group. A high urine pH in patients who present with radiolucent stones provides an additional clue, as uric acid stones develop in acidic urine. In addition, APRT deficiency should always be included in the differential diagnosis of childhood acute kidney injury, especially when associated with radiolucent kidney stones diagnosed by imaging techniques. The pathognomonic round and brown DHA crystals can usually be detected by urine microscopy in non-oliguric patients. Another clue for the identification of DHA crystals is a central Maltese cross pattern that can be observed when small- or medium-sized crystals are viewed by polarized light microscopy (Figure 6.2). [39] Furthermore, analysis of DHA crystals and stone material easily differentiates DHA from uric acid and xanthine. Absence of APRT activity in red cell lysates is diagnostic of APRT deficiency. Enzyme activity measurements are also needed to determine the functional significance of novel mutations. Identification of functionally significant mutations in both copies of the APRT gene confirms the diagnosis. Renal histological examination will reveal DHA crystalline nephropathy in patients with APRT deficiency and CKD or acute allograft dysfunction, even in the absence of a kidney stone history. [94] An outline of the diagnostic algorithm for APRT is presented in Figure 6.3.

6.7. Treatment

Treatment with the XDH inhibitor allopurinol is effective and generally well tolerated in patients with APRT deficiency. Allopurinol 5-10 mg/kg/day, taken either as a single dose or divided into two doses, prevents stone formation, renal crystal deposition and the development of kidney failure. [95] Low purine diet and ample fluid intake provide adjunctive benefits to pharmacologic therapy.

6.8. Prognosis

Preventing serous consequence such as CKD is dependent on early recognition of the disease and instituting preventive measures like Low purine diet and ample fluid intake in addition to allopurinol therapy

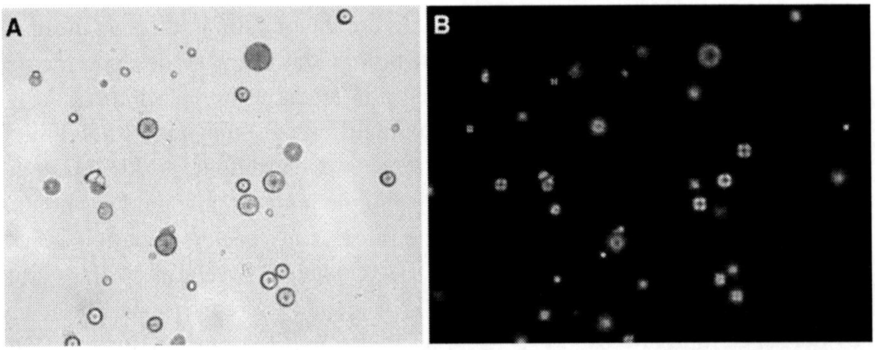

Figure 6.2. Urinary dihydroxyadenine (DHA) crystals. A. Typical small- and medium-sized DHA crystal aggregates (brown with dark outline). B. The same field viewed with polarized light microscopy (yellow in color and produce a central Maltese cross pattern). Diagram from Reference. [39].

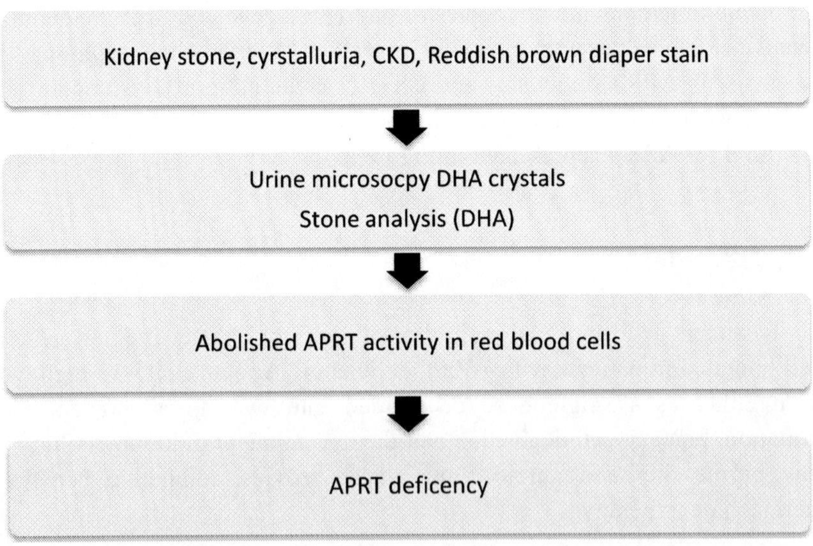

Figure 6.3. Diagnostic algorithm for APRT (adenine phosphorribosyltransferase). DHA (2,8-dihydroxyadenine).

6.9. Conclusion

Adenine phosphoribosyltransferase (APRT) deficiency is a rare inborn error of adenine metabolism resulting in formation of Dihydroxyadenin (DHA) stones, which if not recognized early in life can lead CKD and crystalline nephropathy. It can be confused with uric acid stones by imaging, however, the high urine pH and the typical crystals seen on urine microscopy can be helpful to diagnosis.

Acknowledgment

I would like to thank Professor Raid Bayomi from department of clinical biochemistry and Professor Allal Auhtit from department of genetics for their critical review of this chapter. Both are from the College of Medicine at Sultant Qaboos University, Oman. Also my thanks to The Research Council of Oman for a sponsorship of my Stone analysis research project and Sultan Qaboos University for using the laboratory facilities and support.

References

[1] Wilmer M. J., Schoeber J. P., van den Heuvel L. P. et al., Cystinosis: Practical tools for diagnosis and treatment. *Pediatr. Nephrol.* 2011; 26: 205–215.

[2] Stamatelou K. K., Francis M. E., Jones C. A. et al., Time trends in reported prevalence of kidney stones in the United States: 1976-1994. *Kidney Int.* 2003; 63: 1817–1823.

[3] Hiatt R. A., Dales L. G., Friedman G. D. et al., Frequency of urolithiasis in a prepaid medical care program. *Am. J. Epidemiol.* 1982; 115: 255-265.

[4] Johnson C. M., Wilson D. M., O'Fallon W. M. et al., Renal stone epidemiology: A 25-year study in Rochester, Minnesota. *Kidney Int.* 1979; 16: 624-631.

[5] Curhan G. C., Willett W. C., Rimm E. B. et al., Family history and risk of kidney stones. *J. Am. Soc. Nephrol.* 1997; 8: 1568-1573.

[6] Mente A., Honey R. J. D., McLaughlin J. R. et al., Ethnic differences in relative risk of idiopathic calcium nephrolithiasis in North America. *JURO* 2007; 178: 1992-7.

[7] Rao P. N., Kavanagh J. P. and Preminger G. M., *Urinary Tract Stone Disease. First edition.* London Dordrecht Heidelberg New York: Springer; 2011.

[8] Atan L., Andreoni C., Ortiz V. et al., High kidney stone risk in men working in steel industry at hot temperatures. *Urology* 2005; 65: 858-861.

[9] Soucie J. M., Thun M. J., Coates R. J. et al., Demographic and geographic variability of kidney stones in the United States. *Kidney Int.* 1994; 46: 893-899.

[10] Jungers P., Joly D., Blanchard A. et al., Inherited monogenic kidney stone diseases: Recent diagnostic and therapeutic advances. *Nephrol. Ther.* 2008; 4: 231-255.

[11] Monico C. G. and Milliner D. S., Genetic determinants of urolithiasis. *Nat Rev Nephrol* 2012; 8: 151-162.

[12] Cameron M. A., Sakhaee K. and Moe O. W., Nephrolithiasis in children. *Pediatr. Nephrol.* 2005; 20: 1587-1592.

[13] Coward R. J. M., Peters C. J., Duffy P. G. et al., Epidemiology of paediatric renal stone disease in the UK. *Arch. Dis. Child.* 2003; 88: 962-965.

[14] Grunfeld J. P., Hereditary renal diseases. *Saudi J Kidney Dis Transpl* 1997; 8: 227-234.

[15] Rule A. D., Bergstralh E. J., Melton L. J. et al., Kidney stones and the risk for chronic kidney disease. *Clin J Am Soc Nephrol* 2009; 4: 804-811.

[16] Jungers P., Joly D., Barbey F. et al., ESRD caused by nephrolithiasis: prevalence, mechanisms, and prevention. *Am. J. Kidney Dis.* 2004; 44: 799-805.

[17] Gambaro G., Favaro S. and D'Angelo A., Risk for renal failure in nephrolithiasis. *Am. J. Kidney Dis.* 2001; 37: 233-243.

[18] Schubert G., Stone analysis. *Urol. Res.* 2006; 34: 146-150.

[19] Al-Hinai A. K., Al-Marhoon M. S. and Bayoumi R., *Urolithiasis in Oman*. Master thesis. Sultan Qaboos University, 2013.

[20] Croppi E., Ferraro P. M., Taddei L. et al., Prevalence of renal stones in an Italian urban population: A general practice-based study. *Urol. Res.* 2012; 40: 517-522.

[21] Gambaro G., Reis-Santos J. M. and Rao N., Nephrolithiasis: Why doesn't our 'learning' progress? *European Urology* 2004; 45: 547-56.

[22] B. H., E. L. and D. M., *Urolithiasis and nephrocalcinosis in childhood.* In: Comprehensive Pediatric Nephrology. Elsevier Health Sciences 2008.

[23] Gambaro G., Vezzoli G., Casari G. et al., Genetics of hypercalciuria and calcium nephrolithiasis: From the rare monogenic to the common polygenic forms. *Am. J. Kidney Dis.* 2004; 44: 963-986.

[24] Ferraro P. M., D'Addessi A. and Gambaro G., When to suspect a genetic disorder in a patient with renal stones, and why. *Nephrol. Dial. Transplant.* 2013; 28: 811-820.

[25] Bittles A. H., Endogamy, consanguinity and community disease profiles. *Community Genet* 2005; 8: 17-20.

[26] Chillarón J., Font-Llitjós M., Fort J. et al., Pathophysiology and treatment of cystinuria. *Nat Rev Nephrol* 2010; 6: 424-434.

[27] Milliner D. S. and Murphy M. E., Urolithiasis in pediatric patients. *Mayo Clin. Proc.* 1993; 68: 241-248.

[28] Knoll T., Zöllner A., Wendt-Nordahl G. et al., Cystinuria in childhood and adolescence: Recommendations for diagnosis, treatment, and follow-up. *Pediatr. Nephrol.* 2005; 20: 19-24.

[29] Beara-Lasic L., Edvardsson V. O. and Palsson R., Genetic causes of kidney stones and kidney failure. *Clinic Rev Bone Miner Metab* 2012; 10:2-18.

[30] Al-Marhoon M. S., Bayoumi R., Al-Farsi Y. et al., *The first study of urinary stone composition in the Sultanate of Oman.* Experts in stone disease, Cape Town. *Urolithiasis* 2014.

[31] Pras E., Arber N., Aksentijevich I. et al., Localization of a gene causing cystinuria to chromosome 2p. *Nat. Genet.* 1994; 6: 415-419.

[32] Fernández E., Carrascal M., Rousaud F. et al., rBAT-b (0,+) AT heterodimer is the main apical reabsorption system for cystine in the kidney. *Am. J. Physiol. Renal Physiol.* 2002; 283: F540-8.

[33] Strologo Dello L., Pras E., Pontesilli C. et al., Comparison between SLC3A1 and SLC7A9 cystinuria patients and carriers: A need for a new classification. *J. Am. Soc. Nephrol.* 2002; 13: 2547-2553.

[34] Strologo Dello L., Laurenzi C., Legato A. et al., Cystinuria in children and young adults: Success of monitoring free-cystine urine levels. *Pediatr. Nephrol.* 2007; 22: 1869-1873.

[35] Martens K., Jaeken J., Matthijs G. et al., Multi-system disorder syndromes associated with cystinuria type I. *Curr. Mol. Med.* 2008; 8: 544-550.
[36] Worcester E. M., Coe F. L., Evan A. P. et al., Reduced renal function and benefits of treatment in cystinuriavs other forms of nephrolithiasis. *BJU Int* 2006; 97: 1285-1290.
[37] StrologoDello L. and Rizzoni G., Cystinuria. *Acta Paediatr Suppl* 2006; 95: 31-33.
[38] Saw K. C., McAteer J. A., Monga A. G. et al., Helical CT of urinary calculi: Effect of stone composition, stone size, and scan collimation. *AJR Am J Roentgenol* 2000;175: 329-332.
[39] Edvardsson V. O., Goldfarb D. S., Lieske J. C. et al., Hereditary causes of kidney stones and chronic kidney disease. *Pediatr. Nephrol.* 2013; 28: 1923-1942.
[40] Goldfarb D. S., Coe F. L. and Asplin J. R., Urinary cystine excretion and capacity in patients with cystinuria. *Kidney Int.* 2006; 69: 1041-1047.
[41] Chow G. K. and Streem S. B., Medical treatment of cystinuria: Results of contemporary clinical practice. *JURO* 1996; 156: 1576-1578.
[42] Pareek G., Steele T. H. and Nakada S. Y., Urological intervention in patients with cystinuria is decreased with medical compliance. *JURO* 2005; 174: 2250-2.
[43] Chow G. K. and Streem S. B., Contemporary urological intervention for cystinuric patients: Immediate and long-term impact and implications. *JURO* 1998; 160: 341-4.
[44] Trinchieri A., Montanari E., Zanetti G. et al., The impact of new technology in the treatment of cystine stones. *Urol. Res.* 2007; 35: 129-132.
[45] Katz G., Lencovsky Z., Pode D. et al., Place of extracorporeal shock-wave lithotripsy (ESWL) in management of cystine calculi. *Urology* 1990; 36: 124-128.
[46] Thorleifsson G., Holm H., Edvardsson V. et al., Sequence variants in the CLDN14 gene associate with kidney stones and bone mineral density. *Nat. Genet.* 2009; 41: 926-930.
[47] Bid H. K., Chaudhary H. and Mittal R. D., Association of vitamin-D and calcitonin receptor gene polymorphism in paediatric nephrolithiasis. *Pediatric Nephrology* 2005; 20:773-6.
[48] Reed B. Y., Gitomer W. L., Heller H. J. et al., Identification and characterization of a gene with base substitutions associated with the

absorptive hypercalciuria phenotype and low spinal bone density. *J. Clin. Endocrinol. Metab.* 2002; 87: 1476-1485.

[49] Chen W. C., Wu H. C., Lu H. F. et al., Calcitonin receptor gene polymorphism: A possible genetic marker for patients with calcium oxalate stones. *European Urology* 2001; 39: 716-719.

[50] Janicic N., Soliman E., Pausova Z. et al., Mapping of the calcium-sensing receptor gene (CASR) to human chromosome 3q13.3-21 by fluorescence in situ hybridization, and localization to rat chromosome 11 and mouse chromosome 16. Mamm. *Genome* 1995; 6: 798-801.

[51] Waldegger S. and Jentsch T. J., From tonus to tonicity: Physiology of CLC chloride channels. *J. Am. Soc. Nephrol.* 2000; 11: 1331-1339.

[52] Devuyst O., Christie P. T., Courtoy P. J. et al., Intra-renal and subcellular distribution of the human chloride channel, CLC-5, reveals a pathophysiological basis for Dent's disease. *Hum. Mol. Genet.* 1999; 8: 247-257.

[53] Piwon N., Günther W., Schwake M. et al., ClC-5 Cl-channel disruption impairs endocytosis in a mouse model for Dent's disease. *Nature* 2000; 408: 369-73.

[54] Yu A. S., Role of ClC-5 in the pathogenesis of hypercalciuria: Recent insights from transgenic mouse models. *Curr. Opin. Nephrol. Hypertens.* 2001; 10: 415-420.

[55] Hoopes R. R., Shrimpton A. E., Knohl S. J. et al., Dent Disease with mutations in OCRL1. *Am. J. Hum. Genet.* 2005; 76: 260-267.

[56] Michelis M. F., Drash A. L., Linarelli L. G. et al., Decreased bicarbonate threshold and renal magnesium wasting in a sibship with distal renal tubular acidosis. (Evaluation of the pathophysiological role of parathyroid hormone). *Metab. Clin. Exp.* 1972; 21: 905-920.

[57] Weber S., Schneider L., Peters M. et al., Novel paracellin-1 mutations in 25 families with familial hypomagnesemia with hypercalciuria and nephrocalcinosis. *J. Am. Soc. Nephrol.* 2001; 12: 1872-1881.

[58] Rodríguez-Soriano J., Vallo A. and García-Fuentes M., Hypomagnesaemia of hereditary renal origin. *Pediatr. Nephrol.* 1987; 1: 465-472.

[59] Simon D. B., Lu Y., Choate K. A. et al., Paracellin-1, a renal tight junction protein required for paracellular Mg2+ resorption. *Science* 1999; 285: 103-106.

[60] Li J., Ananthapanyasut W. and Yu A. S., Claudins in renal physiology and disease. *Pediatr. Nephrol.* 2011, 26. 2133-2142.

[61] Alper S. L., Genetic diseases of acid-base transporters. *Annu Rev Physiol* 2002; 64:899-923

[62] Stover E. H., Borthwick K. J., Bavalia C. et al., Novel ATP6V1B1 and ATP6V0A4 mutations in autosomal recessive distal renal tubular acidosis with new evidence for hearing loss. *J Med Genet.* 2002; 39: 796-803.

[63] Frymoyer P. A., Scheinman S. J., Dunham P. B. et al., X-linked recessive nephrolithiasis with renal failure. *N. Engl. J. Med.* 1991; 325: 681-686.

[64] Frishberg Y., Dinour D., Belostotsky R. et al., Dent's disease manifesting as focal glomerulosclerosis: Is it the tip of the iceberg? *Pediatr. Nephrol.* 2009; 24: 2369-2373.

[65] Konrad M., Schaller A., Seelow D. et al., Mutations in the tight-junction gene claudin 19 (CLDN19) are associated with renal magnesium wasting, renal failure, and severe ocular involvement. *Am. J. Hum. Genet.* 2006; 79: 949-957.

[66] Godron A., Harambat J., Boccio V. et al., Familial hypomagnesemia with hypercalciuria and nephrocalcinosis: Phenotype-genotype correlation and outcome in 32 patients with CLDN16 or CLDN19 mutations. *Clin J Am Soc Nephrol* 2012; 7: 801-809.

[67] Brenner R. J., Spring D. B., Sebastian A. et al., Incidence of radiographically evident bone disease, nephrocalcinosis, and nephrolithiasis in various types of renal tubular acidosis. *N. Engl. J. Med.* 1982; 307: 217-221.

[68] Stechman M. J., Loh N. Y. and Thakker R. V., Genetic causes of hypercalciuric nephrolithiasis. *Pediatr. Nephrol.* 2009; 24: 2321-2332.

[69] Praga M., Vara J., González-Parra E. et al., Familial hypomagnesemia with hypercalciuria and nephrocalcinosis. *Kidney Int.* 1995; 47: 1419-1425.

[70] Cebotaru V., Kaul S., Devuyst O. et al., High citrate diet delays progression of renal insufficiency in the ClC-5 knockout mouse model of Dent's disease. *Kidney Int.* 2005; 68: 642-652.

[71] Lieske J. C., Spargo B. H. and Toback F. G., Endocytosis of calcium oxalate crystals and proliferation of renal tubular epithelial cells in a patient with type 1 primary hyperoxaluria. *JURO 1*992; 148: 1517-1519.

[72] Hoppe B., Beck B. B. and Milliner D. S., The primary hyperoxalurias. *Kidney Int.* 2009; 75: 1264-1271.

[73] Coulter-Mackie M. B., Preliminary evidence for ethnic differences in primary hyperoxaluria type 1 genotype. *Am. J. Nephrol.* 2005; 25: 264-268.

[74] Danpure C. J., Molecular etiology of primary hyperoxaluria type 1: new directions for treatment. *Am. J. Nephrol.* 2005; 25: 303-310.

[75] Milliner D. S., The primary hyperoxalurias: an algorithm for diagnosis. *Am. J. Nephrol.* 2005; 25: 154-160.

[76] Belostotsky R., Seboun E., Idelson G. H. et al., Mutations in DHDPSL are responsible for primary hyperoxaluria type III. *Am. J. Hum. Genet.* 2010; 87: 392-399.

[77] Monico C. G., Rossetti S., Olson J. B. et al., Pyridoxine effect in type I primary hyperoxaluria is associated with the most common mutant allele. *Kidney Int.* 2005; 67: 1704-1709.

[78] Milliner D., Treatment of the primary hyperoxalurias: a new chapter. *Kidney Int.* 2006; 70: 1198-1200.

[79] Leumann E., Hoppe B. and Neuhaus T., Management of primary hyperoxaluria: efficacy of oral citrate administration. *Pediatr. Nephrol.* 1993; 7: 207–211.

[80] Hoppe B., Groothoff J. W., Hulton S-A. et al., Efficacy and safety of Oxalobacterformigenes to reduce urinary oxalate in primary hyperoxaluria. *Nephrol. Dial. Transplant.* 2011; 26: 3609-3615.

[81] Pais V. M. Jr., Lowe G., Lallas C. D. et al., *Xanthine urolithiasis. Urology* 2006; 67: 1084e9-11.

[82] S., S. R. and T. N., H*ereditary xanthinuria.* In: The Metabolic & Molecular Bases of Inherited Disease. New York; Montreal: McGraw-Hill 2001.

[83] Levartovsky D., Lagziel A., Sperling O. et al., XDH gene mutation is the underlying cause of classical xanthinuria: A second report. *Kidney Int.* 2000; 57: 2215-2220.

[84] Gok F., Ichida K. and Topaloglu R., Mutational analysis of the xanthine dehydrogenase gene in a Turkish family with autosomal recessive classical xanthinuria. *Nephrol. Dial. Transplant.* 2003; 18: 2278-2283.

[85] Ankem M. K., Glazier D. B. and Barone J. G., Lesch-Nyhan syndrome presenting as acute renal failure secondary to obstructive uropathy. *Urology* 2000; 56: 1056.

[86] Brock W. A., Golden J. and Kaplan G. W., Xanthine calculi in the Lesch-Nyhan syndrome. *JURO* 1983; 130: 157-159.

[87] Edvardsson V., Palsson R., Olafsson I. et al., Clinical features and genotype of adenine phosphoribosyltransferase deficiency in iceland. *Am. J. Kidney Dis.* 2001; 38: 473-480.

[88] Kelley W. N., Levy R. I., Rosenbloom F. M. et al., Adenine phosphoribosyltransferase deficiency: a previously undescribed genetic defect in man. *J. Clin. Invest.* 1968; 47: 2281-2289.

[89] Broderick T. P., Schaff D. A., Bertino A. M. et al., Comparative anatomy of the human APRT gene and enzyme: nucleotide sequence divergence and conservation of a nonrandom CpG dinucleotide arrangement. *Proc. Natl. Acad. Sci. U. S. A.* 1987; 84: 3349-3353.

[90] Sahota A., Chen J., Boyadjiev S. A. et al., Missense mutation in the adenine phosphoribosyltransferase gene causing 2,8-dihydroxyadenine urolithiasis. *Hum. Mol. Genet.* 1994; 3: 817-818.

[91] Greenwood M. C., Dillon M. J., Simmonds H. A. et al., Renal failure due to 2,8-dihydroxyadenine urolithiasis. *Eur. J. Pediatr.* 1982; 138: 346-349.

[92] Chiba P., Zwiauer K. and Müller M. M., Characterization of an adenine phosphoribosyltransferase deficiency. *Clin. Chim. Acta* 1988; 172: 141-147.

[93] Harambat J., Bollée G., Daudon M. et al., Adenine phosphoribosyltransferase deficiency in children. *Pediatr. Nephrol.* 2012; 27: 571-579.

[94] Nasr S. H., Sethi S., Cornell L. D. et al., Crystalline nephropathy due to 2,8-dihydroxyadeninuria: An under-recognized cause of irreversible renal failure. *Nephrol. Dial. Transplant.* 2010; 25: 1909-1915.

[95] Bollée G., Dollinger C., Boutaud L. et al., Phenotype and genotype characterization of adenine phosphoribosyltransferase deficiency. *J. Am. Soc. Nephrol.* 2010; 21: 679-688.

In: Urolithiasis
Editor: Joseph Fletcher
ISBN: 978-1-63463-500-4

Chapter 5

Surgical Management of Paediatric Urolithiasis

Hosni Khairy Salem
Urology Department, Kasr Alainy School of Medicine,
Faculty of Medicine, Cairo University, Egypt

Abstract

The management of paediatric stone disease has undergone a dramatic evolution in recent times. Over the past two decades, surgical management of urolithiasis in children has developed significantly. Shock wave lithotripsy (SWL) is currently the procedure of choice in treating most upper tract calculi in paediatric urolithiasis. In a growing number of centres, the use of ureteroscopy (URS) has dramatically increased, and is now the first choiceapproach for upper tract stones. Percutaneous nephrolithotomy (PCNL) has replaced open surgical techniques for the treatment of large stone burdens greater than 2 cm in size, with efficacy and complication rates similar to those of the adult population. Recently, laparoscopy and robotic techniques have become an option in the management of paediatric urolithiasis.

This chapter will focus on recent advances in the surgical management of paediatric stone disease.

Chapter Outline:

- Overview of the management of paediatric stones
- Shock wave lithotripsy
- Percutaneous nephrolithotomy
- Ureteroscopy
- Laparoscopic and robotic-assisted pyelolithotomy

Introduction

The prevalence of paediatric urolithiasis has a wide geographical variation, with a prevalence of 5-15% in the developing countries and 1-5% in the developed countries, particularly India, Turkey and Pakistan. This difference may be attributed to genetic, dietary and socioeconomic factors [1].

Problems in the developing countries include delayed presentation with a large stone burden, presentation with renal failure, non-compliant patients, socioeconomic issues and limited resources [2]. The overall goals of the management of paediatric urolithiasis include the prevention of kidney damage (preservation of renal function), pain management, complete clearance of the stones and prevention of new stone formation [2].

The selection of a particular modality for paediatric stone management will depend on the stone site, size, composition (HU unit), anatomic abnormalities, presence of obstruction and/or infection, and the availability of resources [3]. The list of management options includes medical expulsive therapy (alpha-adrenergic blockers), shock wave lithotripsy (SWL), endourological procedures and open surgery [4, 5].

No standardized rules for paediatric stone management have been established due to the absence of prospective randomized studies comparing the different modalities of treatment, besides the vast difference in the available resources between different countries around the world [3].

I. Management of Renal Calculi in Paediatric Age Group

a) Shock Wave Lithotripsy (SWL)

This is the treatment modality for all renal stones 1-2 cm in diameter, with HU unit less than 900, and where there is an absence of infection, uraemia and anatomic abnormalities [6].

The paediatric ureter is more elastic and more distensible than the adult one, which facilitates the passage of stone fragments [6].

The safety and long-term squeal of SWL in paediatric urolithiasis is not clearly defined [7].

In one study that included 84 children, the GFR calculated using 99m Tc-DTPA returned to the pre-SWL values at 3m postoperatively [8]. In another study that included 63 children, follow up at 4m showed no difference in renal scaring, blood pressure or renal failure [9].

In children, concerns remain regarding ionizing radiation and the potential for cancer, especially with repeated treatment (latent radiation-induced cancer). Children are more susceptible than adults to ionizing radiation exposure, since they have a greater population of dividing cells [9].

The safety of radiation exposure has been raised in another study, which was comparable to other radiological studies such as VCUG (10). Moreover, animal studies showed no long-term damage to the female reproductive organs after SWL [11].

The first case of successful SWL in children was reported in 1986 [12].

The success rate and stone clearance will depend on the stone burden and the composition of the stone (HU unit) [12].

HM3 (electrohydraulic) and PiezoLith (piezoelectric) devices had comparable stone-free rates for renal pelvic stones, according to the study by Brinkman and colleagues, with 80% stone-free rate (SFR) for HM3 devices and 72% for PiezoLith devices. Electromagnetic devices are more commonly used in recent years [9].

For calyceal stones, one study found that the calyceal anatomy has no effect on the stone clearance, while in another study, the infundibulo pelvic angle and infundibular length had a significant effect on the SFR [13].

For staghorn stones, the results of SWL are variable (33-83%), with many shortcomings including multiple sessions, anaesthesia, need for ancillary procedures, and ureteral stenting [14, 15].

About one-third of clinically insignificant residual fragments (CISF) has been reported to grow within 24-48 months post-SWL and can be a source of stone formation [16, 17].

The morbidity of SWL in children is minimal, and the complication list includes bruising, ecchymosis, perirenal haematoma, renal colic, stein stresses, arrhythmia, lung injury, haematuria, ureteral obstruction and sepsis. The last two complications may necessitate percutaneous drainage and/or stenting [18].

The complications will increase with a large stone burden (more than 700 mm^3) [18].

All cases should receive general anaesthesia; however, in some centres, if the child is over 12 years old, he or she can receive patient-controlled analgesia, dissociative anaesthesia or intravenous sedation [18].

The localization method includes ultrasound of fluoroscopy [19].

Traditionally, SWL is performed "gated," whereby the lithotripsy rate is synchronized to the electrocardiogram. However, within the last decade, the use of ungated lithotripsy with a fixed rate has also been shown to be safe and efficacious in children. Salem and colleagues evaluated the delivery rate of ungated SWL (80 and 120 shock waves per minute) for paediatric renal stones. They demonstrated that a slow delivery rate of SWL has a greater rate of stone clearance, requiring a lower frequency of secondary procedures and resulting in fewer failed procedures [19].

b) Percutaneous Nephrolithotomy (PCNL)

The main indications for PCNL in children include large stone burden (more than 20 mm), hard stonesof more than 900 HU, significant renal obstruction, renal failure, significant residual stones after open surgery, contraindications to SWL and failure of SWL. PCNL can be used as a monotherapy or a sandwich technique as an adjuvant to SWL. The stone burden will necessitate 3D CT to determine the exact size of the stone. The first reported paediatric PCNL was by Woodhouse and colleagues in 1985 [20].

Concerns about PCNL in children include long-term renal damage, the small kidney size, risk of bleeding and risk of radiation exposure.

Previous studies reported no or minimal scarring on long-term follow-up after PCNL in the paediatric age group [21, 22].

Intraoperative bleeding will depend on the size of the instruments and the number of the tracts used [23, 24].

Management of paediatric renal stones has changed dramatically in the last decade, due to recent advances in technology, instrument manufacture, and new intracorporeal lithotripsy techniques [24, 25].

To avoid hypothermia, a warm blanket should be used to cover the parts of the body that are not in the operative field, reducing the time of operation as much as possible, or the operation can be staged for another session [25].

Recent advances include smaller nephroscopes with an 11-15 Fr access sheath, ultrasound-guided puncture instead of fluoroscopy, availability of

YAG laser, smaller probes for the lithoclast, and ultrasonic disintegration [25-27].

Dilatation can be done either by balloon dilatation or Amplatz Alken dilators.

The list of complications includes bleeding and blood transfusion, injury to the pelvicalyceal system, injury to the nearby organs, sensitivity to ionizing irradiation, failed puncture, sepsis, residual stone, leakage and urinoma, conversion to open surgery, and hypothermia if the operation is prolonged [27].

A two-session approach (the first to establish the tract and the second for stone clearance) has been advised to minimize bleeding."Mini-perc" has been reported with the use of a dilator and a sheath together, which are rapidly introduced into the kidney with minimal morbidity.

c) Laparoscopy

Laparoscopy can replace open surgery in experienced hands.

In one study, Cascale el al. reported on retroperitoneal laparoscopic pyelolithotomy in a paediatric age group who had a large stone burden with previous PCNL failure. Stones in the renal pelvis were removed with intracorporeal closure of the pelvis, and flexible cystoscopy was used for calyceal stones [28]. In another study, Gaur et al. reported on retroperitoneal laparoscopy for impacted stones in the upper ureter, with a 100% success rate and a mean hospital stay of 24 hours [29].

d) Robotic-Assisted Laparoscopic Pyelolithotomy

Lee andcolleagues reported on five patients who underwent robotic-assisted laparoscopic pyelolithotomy. Four patients had staghorn stones and one patient had pelviureteric junction obstruction in addition to the pelvic stones. After pyelotomy, the stones were removed by flexible cystoscope through the robotic port, or the robotic grasper was used. All patients needed stenting. The mean operative time was 315 min, bleeding was minimal (mean 19.0ml), and the mean hospital stay was 3.8 days.

One case was converted to open surgery, while three out of the four remaining cases were rendered stone-free. One case had a 6 mm residual stone in the lower pole [30].

e) Open Surgery

The main indications for open surgery in paediatric renal stones include the presence of congenital abnormalities (PUJO), large stone burden, infective stones, and staghorn stone, particularly in the absence of endourological facilities [31, 32]. The indications are far more common in developing countries (14 %) than in developed countries (0.5-5.4%) [33].

Anatrophic nephrolithotomy was done successfully in 11 patients with minimal morbidity, according to the study of Assimos el al. [34].

II. Management of Ureteral Calculi in Paediatric Age Group

a) Shock Wave Lithotripsy (SWL)

Stones less than 3mm in the distal ureter will pass spontaneously, while stones more than 4mm will likely require treatment in the form of SWL or Ureteroscopy (URS) [35].

Stones smaller than 10mm have a 100 % success rate after SWL, regardless of the location. Stones larger than 10mm in the upper ureter had success rates of 67-78% [36, 37].

The success rate will be much lower for distal stones compared with URS [38].

Shock wave lithotripsy is not suitable for cystine stones, calcium oxalate monohydrate stones, impacted stones, anatomic abnormalities or difficult localization [39-42].

b) Ureteroscopy (URS)

Ureteroscopy has become more popular for the management of paediatric ureteral stones after the advent of smaller-sized URS (4.5F) and flexible URS (6.9F), in addition to small laser fibres (Ho-YAG) [43].

Dilatation of the ureter up to 15 Fr is safe, with no risk of vesico-ureteric reflux or stricture formation. The access sheath has the advantagesof being able to repeatedly access the ureter rapidly with minimal trauma [43, 44].

Stone fragmentation may be accomplished by laser, ultrasonic, pneumatic, lithoclast, or electrohydraulic means. The advantages of the laser are that it produces small fragments of 2-3mm in diameter that can pass spontaneously, and the short depth of penetration (4mm). Laser fibre should be in contact with the stone for proper fragmentation, and the initial setting should be 0.6-0.7 joules at 8-10 hertz [45].

Ultrasonic lithotripsy uses a rigid metal vibrating probe with simultaneous suction, and it is not effective for cystine or calcium oxalate monohydrate stones. Pneumatic or ballistic lithotripsy uses a 2.4 Fr metal probe working as a mechanical hammer [46-48].

The lithoclast is a combination of the ultrasonic and the pneumatic, with more effective fragmentation and shorter operative time [46-48].

Electrohydraulic lithotripsy uses a coaxial flexible probe (1.6-5Fr), but nowadays it is not used due to the risk of ureteral or bladder perforation [46-48].

The extraction devices include the Nitinol Dormia, whether helical tip or zero tip, the three-pronged grasper and the rat-tooth (alligator) forceps [46-84].

The complication list includes vesico-ureteric reflux up to 15% (usually grade I), pain, leakage, ureteral perforation (1.4%), bleeding, conversion to open surgery and residual stones. Most series advise stenting following URS [49-51].

III. Management of Urinary Bladder Calculi in Paediatric Age Group

Bladder stones in the paediatric age group can be managed by the transurethral approach, the percutaneous suprapubic approach, or by open surgery. Transurethral is safe for stones less than 10 mm in diameter. The percutaneous approach can be done using a 26 F nephroscope to save time in the operation. Open cystolithotomy is an option for multiple bladder stones, or for very large bladder stones when endourological facilities are not available. The drawbacks of open surgery include prolonged hospitalization, prolonged catheterization, more analgesia and the risk of scar formation [52].

Management of paediatric urolithiasis is a challenge for the urologist.

Randomized controlled trials comparing different modalities are recommended to reach a consensus regarding the most effective primary treatment modality.

References

[1] Milliner D. S., Murphy ME. Urolithiasis in pediatric patients. *Mayo Clin. Proc.,* 1993; 68:241–8. [PubMed]

[2] Coward R. J., Peters C. J., Duffy P. G., Kellet M. J., Choong S., van't Hoff W. G. Epidemiology of paediatric renal stone disease in the UK. *Arch. Dis. Child.*, 2003;88:962–5. [PMC free article] [PubMed]

[3] Salem H. K., Morsi H. A., Omran A., Daw M. Tubeless PCNL in children. *JPU*, 2007;3(3): 235-8.

[4] Erturhan S., Bayark O., Sarica K., et al. Efficacy of medical expulsive treatment with doxazosin in pediatric patients. *Urology,* 2013; 51(3): 640-3.

[5] Aydogdu O., Burgu B., Gucuk A., et al. Effectiveness of doxazosin in treatment of distal ureteral stonein children. *J. Urol.,* 2009 Dec. ;182(6): 2880-4.

[6] Gofrit O. N., Pode D., Meretyk S., et al. Is the pediatric ureter as efficient as the adult ureter in transporting fragments following ESWL for renal calculi larger than 10 mm? *J. Urol*., 2001; 166:1862-4.

[7] Fayad A., El Sheikh M. G., Abdel Mohsen M., et al. Evaluation of the renal function in children undergoing ESWL. *J. Urol*., 2010; 184: 1111-4.

[8] Vlajkovic M., Slavkovic A., Radovanovic M., Siric Z., Stefanovic V., Perovic S. Long-term functional outcome of kidneys in children with urolithiasis after ESWL treatment. *Eur. J. Pediatr. Surg.,* 2002; 12:118–23. [PubMed

[9] Brinkmann O. A., Griehl A., Kuwertz-Broking E., Bulla M., Hertle L. Extracorporeal shock wave lithotripsy in children. Efficacy, complications and long-term follow-up. *Eur. Urol*., 2001; 39: 591–7. [PubMed]

[10] Kroovand R. L. Pediatric urolithiasis. *Urol. Clin. North Am.,* 1997;24: 173–84. [PubMed]

[11] McCullough D. L., Yeaman L. D., Bo W. J., et al. Effect of shock wave on the rat ovary. *J. Urol.,* 1989;141:666-9.

[12] Newman D. M., Coury T., Lingeman J. E., Mertz J. H., Mosbaugh P. G., Steele R. E., et al. Extracorporeal shock wave lithotripsy experience in children. *J. Urol.,* 1986;136:238–40. [PubMed]

[13] Tan A. H., Al-Omar M., Watterson J. D., Nott L., Denstedt J. D., Razvi H. Results of shockwave lithotripsy for pediatric urolithiasis. *J. Endourol.*, 2004; 18:527–30. [PubMed]

[14] Al-Busaidy S. S., Prem A. R., Medhat M. Pediatric staghorn calculi: The role of extracorporeal shock wave lithotripsy monotherapy with special reference to ureteral stenting. *J. Urol.*, 2003; 169:629–33. [PubMed]

[15] Wang L. J., Wong Y. C., Chuang C. K., Chu S. H., Chen C. S., See L. C., et al. Predictions of outcomes of renal stones after extracorporeal shock wave lithotripsy from stone characteristics determined by unenhanced helical computed tomography: A multivariate analysis. *Eur. Radiol.,* 2005; 15:2238–43. [PubMed]

[16] Afshar K., McLorie G., Papanikolaou F., Malek R., Harvey E., Pippi-Salle J. L., et al. Outcome of small residual stone fragments following shock wave lithotripsy in children. *J. Urol.*, 2004; 172:1600–3. [PubMed]

[17] Nijman R. J., Ackaert K., Scholtmeiier R. J., Lock T. W., Schroder F. H. Long-term results of extracorporeal shock wave lithotripsy in children. *J. Urol.*, 1989; 142:609–11. [PubMed]

[18] Ather M. H., Noor M. A. Does size and site matter for renal stones up to 30-mm in size in children treated by extracorporeal lithotripsy? *Urology,* 2003; 61:212–5. [PubMed]

[19] Salem H. K., Fathy H., El Fayoumy H., et al. Slow versus rapid delivery rate SWL for pediatric renal urolithiasis: A prospective randomized study. *J Urol.,* 2014;19(5):1370-4.

[20] Woodside J. R., Stevens G. F., Stark G. L., Borden T. A., Ball W. S. Percutaneous stone removal in children. *J. Urol.,* 1985;134:1166–7. [PubMed]

[21] Mor Y., Elmasry Y. E., Kellet M. J., Duffy P. G. The role of percutaneous nephrolithotomy in the management of pediatric renal calculi. *J. Urol.,* 1997;158:1319–21. [PubMed]

[22] Dawaba M. S., Shokeir A. A., Hafez A. T., Shoma A. M., El-Sherbiny M. T., Mokhtar A., et al. Percutaneous nephrolithotomy in children: Early and late anatomical and functional results. *J. Urol.,* 2004; 172: 1078–81. [PubMed]

[23] Desai M. R., Kukreja R. A., Patel S. H., Bapat S. D. Percutaneous nephrolithotomy for complex pediatric renal calculus disease. *J. Endourol.*, 2004;18:23–7. [PubMed]

[24] Zeren S., Satar N., Bayazit Y., Bayazit A. K., Payasli K., Ozkeceli R. Percutaneous nephrolithotomy in the management of pediatric renal calculi. *J. Endourol.*, 2002;16:75–8. [PubMed]

[25] Helal M., Black T., Lockhart J., Figueroa T. E. The Hickman peel-away sheath: Alternative for pediatric percutaneous nephrolithotomy. *Endourol.,* 1997;11:171–2. [PubMed]

[26] Jackman S. V., Hedican S. P., Peters C. A., Docimo S. G. Percutaneous nephrolithotomy in infants and preschool age children: Experience with a new technique. *Urology,* 1998;52:697–701. [PubMed]

[27] Desai M., Ridhorkar V., Patel S., Bapat S., Desai M. Pediatric percutaneous nephrolithotomy: Assessing impact of technical innovations on safety and efficacy. *J. Endourol.*, 1999;13:359–64. [PubMed]

[28] Casale P., Grady R. W., Joyner B. D., Zeltser I. S., Kuo R. L., Mitchell M. E. Transperitoneal laparoscopic pyelolithotomy after failed percutaneous access in the pediatric patient. *J. Urol.,* 2004;172:680–3. [PubMed]

[29] Gaur D. D. Retroperitoneal laparoscopic ureterolithotomy. *World J. Urol.,* 1993;11:175–7. [PubMed]

[30] Lee R. S., Passerotti C. C., Cendron M., et al. Early results of robotic assisted laparoscopic lithotomy in adolescents. *J. Urol.,* 2007 Jun.; 177(6): 2306-9.

[31] Paik M. L., Resnick M. I. Is there a role for open stone surgery? *Urol. Clin. North Am.*, 2000;27:323–31. [PubMed]

[32] Sakkas G., Becopoulos T., Karayannis A., Drossos G., Giannopoulou K. Enzymatic evaluation of renal damage caused by different therapeutic procedures for kidney stone disease. *Int. Urol. Nephrol.*, 1995;27:669–77. [PubMed]

[33] Zargooshi J. Open stone surgery in children: Is it justified in the era of minimally invasive therapies? *BJU Int.*, 2001; 88:928–31. [PubMed]

[34] Assimos D. G., Boyce W. H., Harrison L. H., McCullough D. L., Hall J. A. Pediatric anatrophic nephrolithotomy. *J. Urol.,* 1985;133:233–5. [PubMed]

[35] Van Savage J. G., Palanca L. G., Andersen R. D., Rao G. S., Slaughenhoupt B. L. Treatment of distal ureteral stones in children: Similarities to the American urological association guidelines in adults. *J. Urol.*, 2000;164:1089–93. [PubMed]

[36] Landau E. H., Gofrit O. N., Shapiro A., Meretyk S., Katz G., Shenfeld O. Z., et al. Extracorporeal shock wave lithotripsy is highly effective for ureteral calculi in children. *J. Urol.*, 2001; 165:2316–9. [PubMed]

[37] De Dominics M., Matarazzo E., Capozza N., Collura N., Caione P. Retrograde ureteroscopy for distal ureteric stone removal in children. *BJU Int.,* 2005; 95:1049–52. [PubMed]

[38] Kapoor R., Solanki F., Singhania P., et al. Safety and efficacy of percutaneous nephrolithotomy in the pediatric population. *J. Endourol.,* 2008 Apr.; 22(4):637-40.http://www.ncbi.nlm.nih.gov/pubmed/ 18338958

[39] Gedik A., Orgen S., Akay A. F., et al. Semi-rigid ureterorenoscopy in children without ureteral dilatation. *Int. Urol. Nephrol.*, 2008;40(1):11-4. http://www.ncbi.nlm.nih.gov/pubmed/17653831

[40] Smaldone M. C., Cannon G. M. Jr., Wu H. Y., et al. Is ureteroscopy first line treatment for pediatric stonedisease? *J. Urol.,* 2007 Nov.; 178(5): 2128-31. http://www.ncbi.nlm.nih.gov/pubmed/17870124

[41] Erturhan S., Yagci F., Sarica K. Ureteroscopic management of ureteral calculi in children. *J. Endourol.*, 2007 Apr.; 21(4):397-400. http:// www.ncbi.nlm.nih.gov/pubmed/17451329

[42] Minevich E., Sheldon C. A. The role of ureteroscopy in pediatric urology. *Curr. Opin. Urol.*, 2006Jul;16(4):295-8.http:// www.ncbi. nlm.nih.gov/pubmed/ 16770131

[43] Caione P., De Gennaro M., Capozza N., Zaccara A., Appetito C., Lais A., et al. Endoscopic manipulation of ureteral calculi in children by rigid operative ureterorenoscopy. *J. Urol.,* 1990;144:484–5. [PubMed]

[44] Shepherd P., Thomas R., Harmon E. P. Urolithiasis in children: Innovations in management. *J. Urol.,* 1988;140:790–2. [PubMed]

[45] Gupta R., Manohar T., Desai M. R. Antegrade flexible ureteroscopy in supine position for impacted multiple ureteric calculi. *Indian J. Urol.,* 2006; 22:139–41.

[46] Casale P., Grady R. W., Joyner B. D., Zeltser I. S., Kuo R. L., Mitchell M. E. Transperitoneal laparoscopic pyelolithotomy after failed percutaneous access in the pediatric patient. *J. Urol.,* 2004; 172: 680–3. [PubMed]

[47] Gaur D. D. Retroperitoneal laparoscopic ureterolithotomy. *World J. Urol.,* 1993;11:175–7. [PubMed]

[48] Van Savage J. G., Palanca L. G., Andersen R. D., Rao G. S., Slaughenhoupt B. L. Treatment of distal ureteral stones in children:

Similarities to the American urological association guidelines in adults. *J. Urol.,* 2000; 164:1089–93. [PubMed]

[49] Hill D. E., Segura J. W., Patterson D. E., Kramer S. A. Ureteroscopy in children. *J. Urol*., 1990; 144:481–3. [PubMed]

[50] Thomas R., Ortenberg J., Lee B. R., Harmon E. P. Safety and efficacy of pediatric ureteroscopy for management of calculus disease. *J. Urol.,* 1993; 149:1082–4. [PubMed]

[51] Schuster T. G., Russell K. Y., Bloom D. A., Koo H. P., Faerber G. J. Ureteroscopy for the treatment of urolithiasis in children. *J. Urol*., 2002; 167:1813–6. [PubMed]

[52] Mishra S. K., Ganpule A., Manohar T., et al. Surgical management of pediatric urolithiasis, *Indian J. Urol*., 2007; 23(4):428-434.

Index

D

E

F

G

H

I

J

K

L

M

N

O

P

Q

R

S

T

U

V

W

X

Y